I Am
More
than
One

I Am More than One

How Women with Dissociative Identity Disorder

Have Found Success in Life and Work

JANE WEGSCHEIDER HYMAN

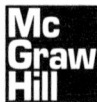

Mc Graw Hill

New York Chicago San Francisco Lisbon London Madrid Mexico City
Milan New Delhi San Juan Seoul Singapore Sydney Toronto

The McGraw·Hill Companies

Library of Congress Cataloging-in-Publication Data

Hyman, Jane Wegscheider.
   I am more than one : how women with dissociated identities have found success
in life and work / Jane Wegscheider Hyman.
        p.   cm.
   Includes biographical references.
   ISBN 0-07-146257-0
   1. Multiple personality.   I. Title.

   RC569.5.M8H96   2007
   616.85'236—dc22   2006016649

1 2 3 4 5 6 7 8 9 0   DOC/DOC   0 9 8 7 6

ISBN-13: 978-0-07-146257-0
ISBN-10:   0-07-146257-0

McGraw-Hill books are available at special quantity discounts to use as premiums and
sales promotions, or for use in corporate training programs. For more information, please
write to the Director of Special Sales, Professional Publishing, McGraw-Hill, Two Penn
Plaza, New York, NY 10121-2298. Or contact your local bookstore.

This book is printed on acid-free paper.

◉

This book is dedicated to the women whose experiences made it possible, and, as always, to JFH and HW.

◉

The I, the I, is what is deeply mysterious.
—*Ludwig Wittgenstein,* Notebooks, 1914–1916

◉

CONTENTS

◉

ACKNOWLEDGMENTS

◉

SO MANY GENEROUS PEOPLE were involved in this book that I would call it a group effort. Of course, my first thanks go to the ten women whose lives are the book's substance. Barbara, Caroline, Ellie, Elizabeth, Gabbi, Lucy, Reba, Samantha, Ruth, and Veronica gave their time for repeated interview sessions and for my follow-up questions on any unclear points. Months or years later, almost all of them critiqued at least one chapter draft, some of them more than one. They are the people to whom I owe the most, and the ones I may not thank by their true, full names.

Each draft of each chapter benefited from comments made by outside readers. Colleagues I met through the Wellesley Centers for Women were excellent critics of chapter drafts and sounding boards for ideas and theories. Among those colleagues, Ruth Hannon and Gina Ogden met with me long after our year at Wellesley for lunchtime critiquing sessions of each other's work. The Wellesley Centers and the Women's Studies Program at Northeastern University each supported this project with a year's affiliation as a visiting scholar.

Researchers and therapists specializing in the effects of traumatic experiences gave their invaluable perspectives on chapter drafts and referred me to research articles I had overlooked. Most of these specialists, whose names are included in the last paragraph, are members of the International Society for the Study of Dissociation and/or the New England Society for the Treatment of Trauma and Dissociation. I benefited from the excellent presentations at the New England Society's meetings as well as from several members' critiques of chapter drafts.

Friends and family members gave me their encouragement and enthusiasm as well as their responses to chapters. Especially Andee Rubin, a friend and excellent editorial critic, spent many evenings with me in a quiet Indian restaurant over discussions of chapter contents with pages spread on the table.

I am also grateful to my agent, Joel Delbourgo, as well as to Paul Stepansky for referring me to Joel. They both believed in the value of this project, and Joel was an interested, sensitive reader who offered suggestions for revisions as well as for contacting publishers and negotiating a contract. I was fortunate in having Judith McCarthy as my editor at McGraw-Hill. She offered perceptive and valuable advice and was enthusiastic and knowledgeable. Her editorial expertise and empathy with the subject were an unsurpassable combination.

My warm thanks to all those I have already mentioned and to those listed alphabetically here: Pat Bishop, Elizabeth Bowman, Caroline Caswell, Jo Anne Citron, Judith Cohen, Philip M. Coons, Michael D. De Bellis, Joanna Duda, Janina Fisher, Fran Grossman, Charles Hyman, Jack Hyman, Susan Miller, Sue Motulsky, Ellert Nijenhuis, Hilda Maria Gaspar Pereira, Cynthia Ritsher, Colin A. Ross, Rhonda L. Sabo, Juliet Sanger, Peggy Schoditsch, Raya Stern, Martin H. Teicher, Joanne H. Twombly, Lynn Wasnak, Sonja Wetzsteon, Sarah Zall.

I Am
More
than
One

INTRODUCTION

Sometimes it was like I could see myself fading. I would be doing something and then I could feel myself being sucked back in a vacuum. And it was like I was standing back watching my body do whatever was going on. Sometimes I would be sucked back in the background and then everything would go black. And when I would come out again I would have to try and figure out, "Is it still the same day, or what day is it, or what time is it?" trying to get myself reoriented and trying at the same time not to let on that I *didn't* know where I was or what day it was.

—*Reba, a thirty-two-year-old nurse*

⊙

THESE ARE THE WORDS of Reba, one of over two and a half million women in the United States who have dissociated parts of the mind. Reba would experience hours, days, or longer in which she was active but afterward could not remember what she did. During the forgotten time, she sometimes discovered herself at night in strange and distant parts of her city and had to call her therapist for help in getting home. Through her supervisor at work, Reba would learn that she had missed several days at her job, days that had disappeared from Reba's memory. Years of therapy have greatly reduced Reba's periodic loss of control over her consciousness. However, she still hears several different voices inside her head speaking to her or to each other, and finds different handwritings in her journal.

Reba is one of the ten women I interviewed who have dissociated parts of the mind. These parts have their own identities, and they alternate control of the body's speech, memory, and action on an almost daily basis. My interviewees are from diverse walks of life and professionally active, but their variations in identity are usually invisible to the outside world. Because of their invisibility, no one knows how many actively professional women are represented among the total number of women who have minds in dissociated parts. Many people believe that such women are found mainly in psychiatric hospitals or intensive outpatient care. My goal was to reveal them as competent professionals, understand the workings of their fascinating minds, capture the quality of their lives, and discover what their uniqueness can teach other people.

The seeds for this book were planted years earlier during my study of women who repeatedly cut, hit, or burn themselves. Several of those women told me they had dissociated states of consciousness that were separate identities. They used various terms for their other identities: "parts," "alter identities," "personalities," "ways," "selves," "my others," and "my people." In this book I most often use the term *parts* to stand for parts of the mind. The self-injuring women explained that sometimes other parts of their minds did the act of self-injury. A woman named Meredith, who repeatedly cut herself with razor blades, told me that she heard voices talking inside her head. Meredith had not told her therapist about the voices, fearful of what they might mean and that her therapist might consider her insane. To a knowledgeable therapist, such voices are an indication to probe more deeply into Meredith's experiences. Questions to ask include:

1. Does she have two or more distinct identities, each with its own pattern of perceiving and relating to the environment and herself?
2. If so, do her identities periodically take control of her body's speech and behavior?
3. Does she experience amnesia that cannot be explained by ordinary forgetfulness?
4. Does she drink alcohol, take any drugs, or have a medical condition that might account for her experiences?[1]

If the answer was yes to the first three questions and no to the fourth, Meredith's therapist might have reassured her that her experiences do not indicate hopeless insanity, but that they are understandable, shared by others, and have a name: *dissociative identity disorder*, or *DID*, formerly known as multiple personality disorder (MPD). Meredith's therapist already knew of the well-documented abuse Meredith had suffered as a child and might have told her that dissociated parts of the mind develop as a result of trauma, especially repeated, interpersonal trauma usually beginning early in life, such as child abuse within the home.

By the time the self-injury project was published,[2] I was beginning a study on the lives of women who share Meredith's experiences. I hoped to erase some of the stigma and correct some misconceptions—including my own—about signs of severe psychological distress as dramatic as having dissociated identities. I use the term *dramatic* because the concept of multiple identities can evoke images of an actress playing a variety of roles in one play. Understandably, one could assume that changes in identity would be noticeable, even blatant, like a skilled actress's change of role. These women taught me why their own identity changes are quite different from those of an actress.

A whole set of assumptions can come with the idea of identity changes. Surely the person must realize that her experiences are unusual; surely all those who know her recognize her many identities; surely therapists can easily identify and correctly diagnose DID; surely a normal family life and a steady job are out of the question; and most certainly a person who has DID wants to have all parts of the mind unified. I originally shared some of these assumptions, although I should have known better, having just had some assumptions about self-injury radically revised by the women I interviewed for that project. With dissociated identities, I had to relearn that listening to the women who have the experiences was going to change my mind. Although some of the assumptions I have listed about having dissociated parts of the mind are true for some people some of the time, their opposite is also often true, as the following chapters will reveal.

Since the 1980s, when a group of interested mental-health professionals rediscovered dissociation, nine times more women than men have been diagnosed as having dissociative identity disorder.[3] This striking disproportion is based on statistics gathered by hospitals and/or psychiatric professionals. More girls are victims of sexual abuse than are boys,[4] a fact that may help explain the imbalance. However, more boys than girls are diagnosed as having DID.[5] Why does this gender ratio in diagnoses change so dramatically by adulthood? One explanation is that many suffering men may avoid seeking help for any mental health problem, seeing therapy as a sign of weakness and an admission of vulnerability discrepant with their views of maleness. Also, men may generally have fewer dissociated parts and fewer outward manifestations than women, making them even more difficult than women to identify. In addition, alcohol and other drugs can be used to dissociate from intolerable memories and feelings, and substance abuse frequently accompanies dissociative identity disorder. Yet, more men than women are diagnosed as alcohol abusers.[6] Possibly more men than women dissociate chemically, while more women than men dissociate psychologically.[7] Or, perhaps men's signs of dissociated identities are more successfully hidden behind substance abuse than are women's signs.

Another explanation is related to men's tendencies to discharge overwhelming feelings, especially rage, through violence. Men abused as children, including men with parts, who are full of shame and rage, are more likely than their female counterparts to react violently to authority figures whose behavior reminds them of their abusers.[8] In prison, they may reenact their childhood entrapment and suffering. Indeed, childhood abuse tends to send women to psychiatric hospitals and men to prison, and in prison settings, men diagnosed as having DID outnumber women.[9] Therefore, the nine to one gender ratio for DID recorded by hospitals, clinics, or private practices might change if incarcerated men could or would seek professional help outside prison.[10]

DID is unique in the field of psychiatry and psychology in that some people, including some therapists, do not think it exists. This denial persists despite more than a century of professional evidence of the phenomenon. Denial should become more difficult, I would think, now that brain imaging techniques can track changing patterns within the brain that match parts of the mind's different senses of self. However, I can understand why DID can be a disturbing concept, one that a person would rather disavow. For, if a person can be a composite of identities, as the following chapters reveal, what does this imply about my own precious sense of self? Personal identity is vital to a feeling of self-worth, and DID threatens the definition of this highly valued concept called "identity."

Social identity is also threatened, because of a basic human need to belong to a group. For many people, the comfort of belonging depends on the ability to distinguish one's own group from groups of people who are "different." Therefore, the other group must be readily identifiable. Active, professional women who have dissociated parts of the mind endanger social identity by blending unnoticeably with the much larger group of people who have none. So, the question arises, how many women who have parts do I know without realizing it? Is such a woman one of my best friends? Have I had an affair with one? Do I work with one? Am I married to one? Am I one? Furthermore, the women I interviewed are the daughters of a college professor, a laborer, a physician, a mechanic, a nurse, and a state government official, among others, and all of these diverse parents are child abusers. If severe, repetitive childhood abuse occurs unnoticed within families of every social status, what does this imply about my own risk of being or becoming an abusive parent? How many child abusers do I know without realizing that I know them? Inadvertently, the women I interviewed challenge personal and social identity in disquieting ways.

Even while DID disquiets, it also fascinates. The very idea of having more than one identity captures the imagination: Can this actually happen? If so, how is it possible? How does someone with several identities behave and feel? Is she like Dr. Jekyll and Mr. Hyde? Is she like film depictions of women who have minds in dissociated parts? To answer such questions, many books have been written, generally by therapists and by people who have parts. Yet, I realized during the self-injury project that women who have parts were telling me things no books or articles had ever mentioned, and their spontaneous accounts raised more questions: "How and why did the various parts of your mind first appear?" "What does it feel like to have one of them take control of the body?" "When they are not in control, how do you know they are there?" "Do you process thoughts and feelings differently from the way I process them?" "How do you make decisions when different parts of your mind have different opinions?" "How are your children affected by the other parts of your mind?" "If you are the part of your mind who is the professional, what happens if another part of your mind takes over while you are at work?" I wanted to see how a woman who has several different states of consciousness functions in a world in which the majority have one state of consciousness and one set of memories. I tried to get inside their heads, and I found there a fascinating, largely unexplored world.

DID affects an estimated 1 percent of adults in the general population of most countries where estimates are available, including the United States, Canada, Belgium, Holland, and Turkey.[11] Data suggest that members of all the largest racial groups and all walks of life are affected.[12] More than two and a half million women in the United States alone are estimated to have dissociated parts,[13] yet almost nothing is publicly known about how having a mind in parts affects these women's lives and the lives of those around them, what their inner world is like, and how they can be better integrated and accepted in a world of minds structured differently from their own.[14]

A woman who has parts generally keeps them a secret, and her secrecy is partly why others know so little about her. She has good reasons for her secrecy. Disclosure can mean losing her job or custody of her children. In the popular view, having parts is synonymous with being "crazy" or unable to function effectively[15] and behaving recognizably differently from the norm. For those who hold such a view, the contents of this book will come as a surprise. Several chapters describe women with structures of the mind vastly different from the norm. An equal number of chapters track these same women through their outwardly mostly unremarkable daily lives as partners, mothers, and grandmothers, and as professionals holding some of the most responsible positions in the workplace, including therapist, nurse, and physician.

My first task for this project was to break through the self-protective secrecy of women who have parts and to find some who were willing to speak openly with me. I required women who had been diagnosed as having DID and who had been working outside the home for several years. Two of the women I had interviewed for the book on self-injury met these requirements and agreed to participate in this project as well. The other participants responded to posted fliers or to advertisements in *Sojourner*, a Massachusetts-based women's newspaper, and in *Many Voices*, a well-established, nationwide newsletter for people who have parts. I interviewed twelve women, and have included eight of these women's experiences throughout the book and in my analyses, and some of two other women's interview material where appropriate. I excluded one woman from my study because I suspected a misdiagnosis of DID. Interviews with two other women revealed that their parts remain mostly inside, giving them a type of dissociation different from that of the other interviewees.[16] One of them, Veronica, has parts who express themselves almost exclusively through writing. I have included some of her experiences in the text. Ruth, the twelfth interviewee, withdrew from the study for personal reasons but allowed me to use some of her interview material.

Because no women of color responded to my advertisements, all study participants are white. They range in age from thirty-two to fifty-seven and in background from working class to middle class. These are women who have insight into their experiences, who are functioning in the workplace, and who feel comfortable enough about having DID to respond to intimate questions about themselves. I chose to interview only women who have steady jobs so that my research could show professional women with DID in action. However, all the women I interviewed have been through times of crisis when functioning was extremely difficult, and four of the eight women have been hospitalized, three of them repeatedly. Nonetheless, my interviewees or participants—as I refer to this group of women throughout the book—represent women usually capable of supporting themselves or of helping to support themselves and their families. They do not necessarily represent a broad spectrum of women who have dissociated parts of the mind.

The interviews took place during meetings with each participant or by long-distance telephone, with each interview taking from four to eight hours, conducted in one-to-two-hour sessions. The taped interviews consisted of responses to open-ended questions. These questions were based on my own and others' prior research and on my pilot study, and I constructed and revised the questions over a period of months. All but one of the women filled out a brief questionnaire on personal and family background, types of therapy she had received, and psychiatric hospitalizations. After analyzing the transcribed interviews for themes and patterns, I edited and rearranged some of them in narrative form so that two chapters are entirely in the women's own voices. Direct quotes are a part of all other chapters. These quotes I combined with my analyses of the most engrossing interview texts I have ever worked with. Drafts of each chapter were then critiqued by at least one of the interviewees as well as by therapists who specialize in dissociative identity disorder, colleagues, and friends.

These women agreed to be interviewed because they felt strong enough to help others by speaking out as "multiples" living in a world of "singletons." As Reba, a thirty-two-year-old nurse, said, "We want to be able to do something good with what we've been through and use it to help other people." Elizabeth, a forty-two-year-old teacher, agreed, even though the thought of the interview was originally "a little scary, but I felt it was important for me. If I can help someone else with my experience through you, it's a good thing." They spoke to me hoping that their published words will empathically introduce them to the outside world, paving the way for more honesty and less secrecy. All busy women, they gave generously of their time and responded bravely to questions even when the answers brought back painful memories. I asked them questions that they had never before answered, and they told of experiences they had never before described.

In alphabetical order, by the names they chose to use for this project, these are the women who shared their stories:

- Barbara is a forty-year-old single social worker who has a full-time position as a therapist. Barbara has a bachelor of arts and a master's degree in social work.

- Caroline is a fifty-seven-year-old accountant working in tax services, now self-employed. Caroline is the married mother of six and grandmother of ten. Other than courses in accounting, Caroline had no formal education after adolescence.

- Elizabeth is a forty-two-year-old teacher in special education with a bachelor of science degree. Elizabeth is a formerly divorced, now partnered* mother of two working toward a master's degree in education.

- Ellie is a forty-three-year-old retail manager and independent beauty consultant. Ellie has a bachelor of arts and is the married mother of two and grandmother of one.

- Gabbi is a forty-two-year-old partnered director of finance and administration specializing in health care, with a bachelor of arts and a master's degree in business administration.

- Lucy is a forty-four-year-old partnered social worker who has a full-time position as a therapist, a private practice, and teaches in a bachelor of art's program for human services. Lucy has a bachelor of arts, a master's degree in music education, and a master's degree in social work. She has two stepchildren.

- Reba is a thirty-two-year-old single registered nurse with a bachelor of science in nursing. Reba is the comother of her niece and nephew, alternating their care with her sister.

- Samantha is a forty-three-year-old lawyer specializing in bankruptcy law. Samantha has a bachelor of arts, a master's degree in library science, and a doctorate in law. She is the divorced mother of twelve and grandmother of one.

---

*Following one of my interviewees' suggestions, I refer to those women who are living with a partner as *partnered*.

These two women allowed me to use their experiences peripherally:

- Ruth is a forty-one-year-old divorced physician who lives with her partner.

- Veronica is a fifty-two-year-old single environmental planner specializing in airport and seaport development.

These women were an unceasing source of surprises as they revealed their inner worlds peopled with numerous parts of their minds who have names, jobs, talents, and character, and who sometimes have elaborate "places of residence" within the mind. The women's attitudes toward the parts of their minds, their experiences within the home, and their ability to achieve professionally without anyone guessing that they have more than one identity were revelations. Surprising to me, too, were my own reactions to their accounts. I would never have guessed, for example, that I could come to envy some of them. Yet, I found myself repeatedly thinking, "I wish *I* could do that!" How practical it would be to be able to shut off all distracting thoughts or feelings at work and be all concentration; to suddenly become fearless and relaxed before a public speaking engagement; to escape from the body while my dentist drills; to have a voice inside to help me behave kindly and wisely. I found that some of my interviewees feel a certain degree of pity for those like me who have to endure uncomfortable situations, feel painful feelings, do all tasks and make all decisions alone, and who have no other parts of their minds to keep them company. I came to understand their pity.

Having to occasionally hold back tears while talking with them, or crying while reading the transcribed interviews, did not surprise me. Because of my interviews with women who injure themselves, I suspected that I would hear or read of horrific childhood experiences, although the sadism sometimes surpassed anything I had heard before.[17] Instead, I was surprised at how often I laughed. My interviewees and I laughed together at certain parts' quirks, at embarrassing situations another part of the mind had caused, or at a friend's or partner's amusing reaction to learning about the existence of other parts. Through their humor, my interviewees revealed their fortitude and lack of self-pity, teaching me more about how to live than I had expected to learn. My interviewees could be anyone's good friend, partner, teacher, doctor, therapist, mother, sister, or colleague without those closest to them learning about their unusual inner worlds or guessing that their minds are in dissociated parts. The following pages reveal their extraordinary lives.

AUTHOR'S NOTE

◉

WHILE ANALYZING INTERVIEW TEXTS and writing this book, I constantly made new discoveries about what it means to have several identities within one body. As my knowledge increased, I struggled to find the appropriate language to honor my interviewees' experiences and convey those experiences accurately to the reader. I initially described each identity just as my interviewees describe them. I wrote, for example, "Louisa is a very bright ten-year-old who likes to read and crochet," conveying the words of my interviewee Reba describing a part of her mind called Louisa. In doing so, I described Louisa as a person separate from Reba. Yet, I needed to indicate that Louisa is a part of Reba's mind, not a tangible person. Accuracy demanded that I change a simple description of Louisa to one more complex: "The part of Reba's mind called Louisa is developmentally ten years old and likes to read and crochet." I had to be faithful to my interviewees' perceptions by using their words as much as possible, yet also find a language to convey the reality of several identities within one body.

I was originally hampered by a lifelong habit of thinking in terms of a unified mind. When I began interviewing, I conceived of each interviewee as, for example, Veronica, a whole personality who also has peripheral identities. This concept was more comfortable to me than admitting to myself that the Veronica I interviewed was herself a part of her mind, albeit perhaps the one most mature and versatile and most often seen by the outside world. Therefore, referring to my interviewees involved verbal modifications because each interviewee's name stands for two entities. "Reba," for example, is the name of Reba as a whole personality including all parts of her mind. Reba is also the name of the particular part of her mind who works as a nurse. An interviewee whose name is Samantha is another example. If I write "Samantha is a lawyer," is that an accurate statement? The part of Samantha's mind called Samantha is not a lawyer and knows nothing about law. The lawyer part of Samantha's mind is called "The Smart One." I realized that I had to differentiate between Samantha as the part of her mind who is ignorant of law and Samantha as a whole personality who is a lawyer.

A further dilemma arose regarding how to refer to the parts of a person's mind such as Louisa or The Smart One. I began by using the terms *alter identities*, or *alters*, only to find that some of the (excellent) readers who critiqued my chapter drafts objected. They found that the term *alters* encouraged me to describe alter identities as tangible people. I then changed the term to *parts*, to stand for "parts of the mind," and have kept that term in the book. I had hardly begun using the term *part*, however, when I had to puzzle over the proper pronoun to use in referring to a part of the mind. A part of something is usually an inanimate object. The dissociated parts of the mind I refer to are not inanimate objects but human identities. Therefore, for this book I write, for example, "The part of her mind *who* works as a nurse." The complexity of my interviewees' minds demanded that I expand my way of thinking and my language to be simultaneously faithful to my interviewees' experiences and accurate.

I

SAMANTHA, OR THE LOGIC OF HAVING DISSOCIATED IDENTITIES

About third grade in school I'd hear voices in my head yelling at me or giving me answers. . . . When I lay down to go to sleep at night I'd hear them telling me what I didn't do right during the day and things that I had to do the next day. It was like listening to myself dissecting my day. . . . Or I wouldn't be able to find my shoes in the morning, and I'd hear a voice telling me where my shoes were; or I'd do something wrong, and I'd hear a voice telling me what I should do to make it better and to fix it.

—*Samantha, a forty-three-year-old lawyer*

◉

Samantha, the daughter of two college professors, is a woman with an extraordinarily full life. Twice divorced, she is the mother of twelve and grandmother of one. Her children range in age from six to twenty-three, and five were still living at home at the time she talked with me. (Four of her children are from her second husband's previous marriage, but Samantha raised them.) Besides raising a dozen children, Samantha has a master's of library science and a juris doctor and is a self-employed lawyer specializing in bankruptcy law. As hobbies she plays the flute, quilts, and embroiders.

15

Since the age of eight, Samantha has heard voices inside her head, an experience she perceived as "thinking loudly." The voices, such as those she described at the beginning of this chapter, have so far remained with her. After years of hearing voices and having periods of time she could not remember, the demands on her as lawyer, wife, and mother became overwhelming. Those demands, together with her lack of consistent memory, led to a life of frantic perplexity: "I couldn't keep track of where I was or what I was doing or what I was supposed to do next. It felt like I was on remote control and somebody else was driving the controls and I was going really, really fast."

After four years of therapy, several suicide attempts, and a misdiagnosis, some of Samantha's inner voices began to speak aloud through Samantha's mouth to her therapist during therapy sessions, hours that Samantha could not remember. Only then was she correctly diagnosed as having dissociated parts of the mind, called in diagnosis *dissociative identity disorder* or *DID*. With her therapist's help, Samantha began to understand the meaning of her internal voices and memory lapses and to become acquainted with the specific names and attributes of the parts of her mind behind each voice. Samantha's mind is in twenty parts, including the part called Samantha, and each part has specific purposes. This chapter introduces mainly the three other parts who, besides Samantha, most often take charge of consciousness and functioning and therefore cause Samantha's memory lapses.

At the beginning of our interview, when I began to learn about Samantha's multifaceted life, I asked myself how a woman can have so many responsibilities, be so accomplished, and yet cope with having a mind in parts. Some details from Samantha's life help answer my question and simultaneously reveal the internal logic of having separated parts of the mind.

SAMANTHA'S PSYCHOLOGICAL ESCAPE

Dissociated means "separate from" or "not associated with" and is a crucial term in understanding Samantha. Dissociation is related in some ways to alterations in consciousness many people experience every day. While in a state of absentmindedness, for example, our conscious minds are detached from the body's actions and we do everyday things without awareness. Relaxation techniques using visualization are a type of purposeful separation of a part of the mind from the body's actual place and circumstances. Dissociation, however, refers to a structural separation of the mind related to trauma[1]: terrifying, inescapable experiences that overwhelm the brain's and central nervous system's usual rhythms of functioning. One of the fundamentals of trauma is the feeling of immobilization[2]: something terrible is about to happen; you cannot escape; and nothing you can do will prevent this terrible thing from happening. What might such a terrible event be? Because all of my interviewees mentioned childhood abuse in the course of the interview, I asked each one to tell or write about a typical day or night in which the abuse occurred. The following account is an example from Samantha's life written by a part of Samantha's mind, with spelling, punctuation, and alternating singular and plural personal pronouns as that part wrote it:

AGE NINE

Woke up being spanked by father for sleeping naked on bed with no sheets. Tried to make bed but had to go down for breakfast. Had to eat soft boiled egg when didn't want to eat. Threw up. Cleaned it up. Left for school without shoes cuz couldn't find them. Mother brought shoes to school later. Teased by class for no shoes. Home, homework. Made dinner with mother. Sat with father while he ate when he got home. Went upstairs to bed. Father followed a few minutes later. Got into bed telling me how much he loved me and how special i was to him. He initiated sexual relations and when I responded he punched us in the stomach telling us we were not supposed to enjoy it, it was only for the guy to enjoy. . . . Sex got the bed wet. He spanked me and stripped off the sheets and left. I went out on the roof to ask god to let me die tonight. i didn't die. it didn't even lightning. went inside. too tired to change sheets. slept.

By the age of nine Samantha wanted to die, and this passage tells why. In one twenty-four-hour period she experienced seven incidents of abuse: physical abuse, humiliation, forced feeding, neglect, incestual sexual abuse, and twice again physical abuse. Her account is written in a circular form, with the last sentence leading directly back to the first: "went inside. too tired to change sheets. slept. Woke up being spanked by father for sleeping naked on bed with no sheets." This form suggests abuse repeated over time, as indeed it was: these or other abusive incidents occurred three to four times weekly for fourteen years. What Samantha described is the problem; this chapter discusses a child's brain's solution to the problem, a solution that later can itself become a problem.

God didn't let Samantha die; therefore she had to find a way to bear living with such trauma. When her body could not escape, Samantha escaped psychologically. She automatically dissociated from the event and perceived the experience as though it were happening to someone else, as she told me during the interview.

> I didn't really realize that this was weird at the time, but [when I was about nine] if I didn't want to be in my bed, I could like get out of my bed and go sit on my dresser next to my doll and still be in bed, and watch myself. . . . [That would happen] when my dad came into the room. I remember I could look over and see myself in bed. But it didn't occur to me, "How could I be in bed and be over here at the same time?" . . . I just thought of it as normal.

Cecelia Emerges

Over time, as the part of her mind called Samantha is repeatedly dissociated from her body, the abused body lying on the bed is controlled by a different part, a part who acquires her own identity and whose role is to bear the sexual abuse and keep it separate from Samantha's memory. This part is one of the inner voices Samantha heard as a child and one whom Samantha, with her therapist's encouragement, has been able to internally speak with and see in her mind's eye. Samantha describes this part:

> She's fourteen and she's—well she's a teenager, that's the best way to describe her [Samantha chuckles]. She gets us in a lot of trouble. . . . Her name used to be "The One Who Performs Sexual Functions." . . . She changed her name to Cecelia. But that was her job and is her job, but she does other things too, like if people want to go shopping at the mall she's the one who goes . . . with them 'cause she likes to shop. . . . She likes to flirt with guys; she likes to talk on the Internet to guys. She's short and she has red, real curly hair; no glasses. She has a little bit of freckles. And she likes wearing just jeans and a T-shirt; she doesn't like shoes.

Cecelia specifically fulfills her job requirements. Selections from my interview with Samantha illustrate this point because Cecelia was the part who spoke with me when I turned the subject to sexual relationships. Cecelia is the part of Samantha's mind responsible for sex and for conversations pertaining to the body, such as sex, illness, or surgery. The following short excerpts are from two different sections in the interview, all of which was conducted by long-distance telephone. In the first section, I had just begun the topic of sex. Because Cecelia has a tone of voice and way of speaking very similar to Samantha's, I did not realize that Samantha had been switched to Cecelia at the first mention of sex. Also, it did not register that she referred to her father as "Samantha's father." I began my questions assuming that I was speaking with the part of Samantha's mind called Samantha, and that she would be telling me about relationships with boyfriends and with her two former husbands.

Q. Does anything come to your mind concerning parts and having sexual relationships?
A. I just did what I was told and nobody else was around. Well . . . that's not really true. There were a couple of other people around: . . . The Whipping Boy and The One Who Feels the Pain were there.

Q. When you say you did what you were told, told by whom?
A. By Samantha's father or whoever.

Q. So you mean when you were being abused.

By the following section of the interview, I knew about the switch because Cecelia had revealed her identity to me.

Q. Was there anything else that you wanted to tell me about those times when you had to do what you were told?
A. They weren't much fun.

Q. Was there some other kind of sexual relationship before your marriage?
A. Well, with Samantha's father and with her brother, and with one guy that we went out on a date with.

Q. So this one man you went out on the date with, how was that?
A. It was fun.

Cecelia shows us the many ways she is ideal for her job. She is an adolescent created by a child's brain to be old enough to take sex. She can have abusive sex without feeling or showing any pain because other dissociated parts called The One Who Feels the Pain and The Whipping Boy act as her assistants, their sole jobs being to feel any pain the body must take and to keep a blank face throughout. Samantha's father and brother are not related to Cecelia; they are just men like all the others. For Cecelia, the term *abuse* has little meaning: sex is simply sex, regardless of person and circumstances. The only way she distinguishes between the years of abuse and a high school date is that the former "weren't much fun," while the latter "was fun."

Because Cecelia and her two accomplices were in charge of taking the childhood incest, they shielded Samantha from the physical pain, overwhelming emotions, and all memory of her father's abusive acts. Cecelia "just did what [she] was told," so that her ready acquiescence may also have prevented even worse harm. Moreover, even though Cecelia is fourteen as opposed to Samantha's forty-two, Cecelia blends in with the older persona so that Samantha's absence is not noticed. I realized that I was speaking with Cecelia only after I asked Samantha if she had always remembered the abuse. Her response was, "Well, I'm Cecelia, so I can remember it. But mostly nobody else remembers it 'cause they weren't there." I am not the only person in Samantha's life who did not realize she was speaking with Cecelia. Samantha has been married twice and, as far as Samantha knows, neither husband noticed that only a part of the woman they married experienced physical intimacy. Moreover, whenever their conversation turned to sex or to anything related to the body, Cecelia was the part who answered, without any listener noticing the difference.

Cecelia is the only part of Samantha's mind who wants the experience of having sex and apparently likes it. When I asked Samantha why she thinks Cecelia wants sex, Samantha replied, "'cause that's her job." However, because her job description entails having sex and doing what she is told, she smoothes the way for one-night stands and for further sexually abusive relationships. After all, sex with an abusive man is what she has always known; why not continue it with any man so inclined? Samantha left her father's house at age seventeen to unwittingly marry such a man. Samantha, the young daughter of abusive parents, is unlikely to have been taught the warning signs of an abusive person, signs that even women raised in nonabusive households often do not learn to detect until major decisions and actions, such as a marriage ceremony, have taken place.

Cecelia's characteristics and job description do not coincide favorably with Samantha's characteristics and the kind of life she desires. Here Samantha, who was divorced from her second husband at the time of the interview, gives two examples of the ways in which Cecelia's behavior conflicts with the life Samantha wants to lead. One example is from the past and one from the present.

IN THE PAST
[A]bout twenty years ago, . . . I was in law school and earning money for law school by sleeping with friends of my husband that he brought home. I didn't know I was doing that, but I would wake up sometimes

and be with somebody that I didn't know. [Then a part] would take over . . . so I'd forget about it. They'd just take me out of the situation.

CURRENTLY

We put an ad in one of the AOL dating things. And so they'll respond to our ad or we'll respond to someone else's ad. . . . Sometimes when it's not me, like if Cecelia answers it and she's very provocative, it makes me upset, 'cause that wasn't what I wanted to do. . . . [So] we keep meeting people on the Internet and then meeting them [in person] and having [sexual] relationships with them. It's frustrating because I don't want to be doing that . . . but Cecelia [does]. . . . [What usually happens is] we'll meet for dinner and then if my kids aren't home, we'll go back to my house or sometimes we'll go back to their house. And then Cecelia usually has sex with them. [If it were up to me alone,] I'd be meeting them but I wouldn't be sleeping with them. There are a couple of them that I like, but I don't know if they're in the relationship just for the sex or if they like me.

As Samantha tells us, she has been used as a prostitute and repeatedly has potentially dangerous, perhaps unprotected sex with strangers. Samantha's goal of having a stable, permanent relationship is sabotaged by Cecelia, who wants only sex. Because of Cecelia, therefore, Samantha forfeits participation in and control over her sexual life, major drawbacks for her ever since she left her father's house. Changing this behavior is one of her goals in therapy. During the time of our interviews, Samantha's therapist helped Samantha and other parts set up an internal committee to be in charge during dates. "We don't want Cecelia to take over and do the whole date."

The Smart One

While Cecelia illustrates a part's role in Samantha's personal life, another part of Samantha's mind gives insight into Samantha's professional accomplishments. This part sprang from a different type of abuse.

AGE THREE

We were learning how to read, and we kept mixing up *Spot* and *Puff*, and it was making my parents really, really mad. Together they yelled at me, and my mother spanked me. Then later that night my father punished me: he beat me and he put things inside me. . . . [This happened] probably about three or four times a week.

AGE EIGHT

[I] had to get A's in school [and did] until in third grade I got a C in handwriting. There were a lot of [consequences from my father], mostly sexual.

As Samantha tells us, at the age of three she was tortured for confusing the names *Spot* and *Puff* and around age eight she was sexually abused for getting a C in handwriting. "Intellectual abuse" is not a term found in the literature on child abuse or on parts, but along with torture and emotional, physical, and sexual abuse, I consider intellectual abuse an appropriate term here because it reflects the resulting separation of part of Samantha's mind for all intellectual pursuits. As Samantha explains, "Anything that has to do with a lecture, an assignment, or somebody telling me that there's something I need to learn, then I know that I'm going to be gone." Samantha is "gone" because another part of her mind, appropriately called The Smart One, is switched into control. The Smart One was described twice during the interviews, the first time in a brief written description that The Smart One wrote herself and the second time in Samantha's words.

THE SMART ONE'S DESCRIPTION

F[emale], 43, in charge of anything that requires intelligence. She is a lawyer and teacher and a librarian.

SAMANTHA'S DESCRIPTION

The Smart One came at about three years old because we were learning how to read and we kept mixing up Spot and Puff. . . . So she came 'cause she was really smart, and she could read it without mixing things up. . . . [S]he's . . . kind of abrupt, and she's a very get-to-the-point kind of person. She can read really, really fast, and she makes very smart, rational-type decisions. She doesn't let emotions get in the way; she just adds up the numbers and comes up with an answer. . . . She's tall and real thin [and] likes suits, mostly mauve-colored stuff. And everybody gets drunk except The Smart One; she never gets drunk. So it doesn't matter how much we drink, she can always drive.

When I brought up the topic of work during the interview, The Smart One responded to my questions. I did not notice the switch. All I perceived was a slight change in Samantha's manner of speaking: she seemed matter-of-fact, almost impatient, unlike her usual gentle self, and I wondered if I had said anything to anger her. Also, I could hear the rustle of papers in the background over the telephone, as though she were trying to do paperwork while talking, something she had never done before. When Samantha started telling me about her legal work, I mentioned to her that I thought she had said she could not remember law school. Her response was, "Samantha doesn't remember law school. This is The Smart One," and she explained that she came out because I was asking questions Samantha could not answer. She came out to be helpful, just as Cecelia came out so that the part of Samantha's mind who knows about sex could answer my questions.

Being smart, focused, fast, and rational are all characteristics designed to help a child overwhelmed by age-inappropriate intellectual demands and the terror of subsequent punishment if she fails. "She doesn't let emotions get in the way" is an understatement. The Smart One, as Samantha later told me, does not feel. However, The Smart One takes care of Samantha's professional life, and having no feelings at all would not be popular at the workplace. The Smart One works with another part called Julia who is all emotion: sweet, sensitive, and empathic. The Smart One and Julia make the perfect couple: one is all intellect, the other all emotion—but they are separate. In spite of their separateness as parts of Samantha's mind, they are linked by shared knowledge. Each one knows what the other is doing so that work can proceed smoothly. The Smart One gave me the following two examples of her professional teamwork with Julia.

About Her Work as a Science Librarian

We got our degree to teach and then Samantha's father wanted us to get a degree in library science. So we got a master's degree in library science and worked at a science library. I did that [with] Julia . . .

Later in Her Life, Referring to Law Practice

I do all the legal work: . . . deciding what needs to be done for the client, putting together the paperwork, telling the client what needs to be done, going to court, talking to the other attorneys on the phone. [Julia does] the hand-holding and being nice to people. I'm more abrupt than Julia is and [clients] might notice that. But they probably wouldn't think it was weird.

The Smart One's descriptions reveal two clues vital to her success as a part of Samantha's mind. The first clue is "they probably wouldn't think it was weird." According to The Smart One, her clients notice only that their lawyer is focused and abrupt while discussing business, but can be gracious and empathic when occasion demands. When The Smart One and Julia were created, they were Samantha's age, and they have matured and aged with the body so that they can perpetually "pass" as Samantha. As far as Samantha knows, nothing about their voices or demeanor was or is perplexing or alarming to others, including Samantha's parents, schoolteachers, husbands, employers, or colleagues. As Samantha told me, "We try not to make it obvious." The second clue to The Smart One's success is displayed in her words "Samantha's father." The Smart One does not consider the man who intellectually abused her as her father. He is Samantha's father, just as none of the men Cecelia has slept with are related to her. Also, Samantha's father's demands did not terrify The Smart One because her intellectual capacities rose to meet those demands and because she is incapable of feeling terror or any other emotion. Furthermore, she did not have to suffer the consequences of possible failure. Those consequences are the domain of Cecelia, The One Who Feels the Pain, and The Whipping Boy. Therefore, for The Smart One, Samantha's father's intellectual abuse was not abuse but simply part of the job for which she came.

Samantha does pay a price, however, for The Smart One's expert protection: she forfeits any role in her own intellectual life. She told me what it is like to be "gone" whenever any intellectual demands are made on her. The experiences she relates here were from the time before her diagnosis—before she knew why she was having such experiences.

FROM HER HIGH SCHOOL YEARS

I would lose time, and I just thought I was daydreaming or that I hadn't been paying attention. In high school . . . my homework would get done and I wouldn't remember doing it; I'd read books and not remember anything about what I'd just read. I could have a paper that I had to write . . . and be really, really tired, too tired to write it, and feel like I was just going to go to sleep, and forget it, and not turn it in. And then all of a sudden it would be four in the morning and the whole paper was sitting there all typed and done. I just figured I wasn't paying attention, that I was just kind of daydreaming and not really thinking about it. I couldn't figure out how I could daydream through writing a paper when I couldn't even remember the book, but I figured, "Oh well." My parents kept telling me I was special and I figured, "Okay, that's part of being special."

FROM HER LAW SCHOOL YEARS

[W]hen I [was] about twenty-three . . . [and] started law school, I wouldn't remember anything about being in class. I'd remember driving to school and going to sit down in class. And then the next thing I knew I'd be leaving the school and driving home. And before each law school exam I'd be really nervous . . . because I had no idea how I could take the test; I didn't know any of the stuff. . . . And then I'd hear a voice in my head saying, "Don't worry about it; just take a deep breath and relax and you won't have to worry about it." So I did—then the test would be over. . . . I just thought it was normal; I just thought it was the way I worked.

Samantha knows that she was a straight-A student without ever having had the experience of being a student, and knows she is a lawyer without ever having had the experience of being in law school or practicing law.

Samantha's Gratitude

Samantha's lack of participation in and control over her intellectual and sexual life is a major negative effect of having The Smart One and Cecelia, with Cecelia's continued power being most troublesome. Against these negatives, however, come protective reasons for having dissociated parts.

• *Samantha lived through her childhood and adolescence.* The women I spoke with repeatedly testify that without other parts to shield them from overwhelming emotions during abuse, they would have committed suicide, become unable to function, or "gone insane."

• *Samantha grew up in a "normal" environment.* So complete was the separation within Samantha's mind that memories of abuse did not begin to seep through to her until age thirty-seven, three years after she began therapy. Therefore, she was not aware of much of her parents' behavior and was oblivious to the inescapable threat of life at home.

• *Samantha has a sexual life and a family.* Wanting to have sex and to be in a sexual relationship is understandably not universal among formerly sexually abused women. However, Samantha first married at age nineteen, and other parts protected her throughout her first marriage and well into her second from any inkling of childhood torture and incest. Therefore, the Samantha part was not conscious of abuse experiences to make her wary of men or of marriage. Samantha is largely able to consciously experience motherhood, which is a major joy and the greatest responsibility she can call her own.

• *She maintains an intellectual life.* Anxiety and learning do not mix well. When in a state of anxiety or terror, the brain is largely or entirely incapable of processing information.[3] If Samantha's mind had been unified, fear of the torture that followed reading mistakes or a poor grade would most likely have made effective learning impossible. Therefore, in order to preserve her capacity to learn, Samantha's mind has a part who cannot feel.

• *She has a profession and is good at it.* Because of The Smart One, Samantha did extremely well in law school and was employed by a first-rate law firm for ten years until the demands of child-rearing forced her to work as a lawyer from her home.

• *Samantha was able to support herself.* She worked full-time and, with the help of child support payments, continues to support herself and her children working part-time from her home. If Samantha had become incapable of learning, she could have spent her life on disability benefits.

   With this information, the question I asked myself at the beginning of the interview with Samantha, How can a woman have so many responsibilities and accomplishments and yet be coping with having a mind in parts? now has an answer. Samantha is able to be fulfilled and accomplished, not in spite of the other parts but because she has them. She said as much herself when answering my question about the most important positive or negative effects in her life of having other parts. This was what she considered the most important positive effect:

> I think that if I didn't have the personality that does all of my law work
> and my schoolwork—'cause she can concentrate really hard and get
> everything done really, really quickly—if I didn't have her I don't think
> I would have accomplished nearly what I have accomplished. And I
> don't think *she* could have done it if she had been bothered by the other
> things that the rest of us worry about. So I guess it gave her more intense
> focus and let me be more accomplished.

The prevailing sentiment Samantha expresses here is gratitude toward The Smart One: "If I didn't have her I don't think I would have accomplished nearly what I have accomplished." But her whole system of dissociated parts is also brought out for applause: "I don't think *she* could have done it if she had been bothered by the other things that the rest of us worry about."

Even at the age of eight, long before Samantha knew what they were, other parts of her mind were trying to help her: giving her answers at school, telling her how to correct something she did wrong, helping her find her shoes in the morning. Their necessary help in the past has sometimes become a hindrance in the present, a common dilemma among women who have minds in parts and a situation Samantha and her therapist are trying to alleviate. Nonetheless, having The Smart One, Julia, and Cecelia has preserved Samantha's ability to grow up in her father's house, have a family of her own, and function in the working world. Samantha has come to understand and appreciate the other parts of her mind, as painful and detrimental as their presences may sometimes be.

TRAUMA AND THE STRUCTURE OF SAMANTHA'S MIND

If Samantha had grown up in nontraumatic circumstances, she would have developed a personality that encompasses all experiences, and while growing up and maturing, her mind would have learned how to make its way and, if possible, to thrive in the environment in which she lived. As the parts of Samantha's mind called The Smart One, Julia, and Cecelia illustrate, because of repeated trauma, Samantha could not develop a united mind that contains all aspects of the mind's usual functions, such as relationships of affection, sexual relationships, intellectual activities, perceptions of all emotions and of physical pain, and perceptions of threat or danger.

By early childhood, Samantha's mind was already being flooded with unbearable events, an experience she shares with all of my interviewees. The childhood abuse my interviewees suffered had, for most of them, already begun by the age of five and generally lasted until they were old enough to live independently. Their experiences support other studies showing that among people with dissociated parts of the mind, abuse begins by age nine for over 90 percent, by age five for over 50 percent, and lasts on average over ten years.[4]

Data from several countries suggest that the majority of people who have dissociated parts of the mind suffered their trauma within the family.[5] My interviewees are no exception. Like Samantha, all their primary abusers were parents, in one case the mother and for all others the father, with the majority also having mothers and other relatives or unrelated people as abusers or colluding in the abuse. When the abuse perpetrator is the adult on whom a child relies for love and protection, the psychological consequences are the most devastating,[6] perhaps especially combined with the youth of the victim and the years' duration of the abuse. The relative impact of each type of abuse—sexual, physical, or emotional abuse or neglect—is a matter of debate[7] and the relative impact appears to be different in girls compared to boys.[8] However, experiencing multiple types of abuse may have a greater impact on a child's overall signs of dissociation than any single type of abuse alone.[9]

Several alterations in the developing brain are linked to prolonged childhood abuse or neglect. These changes include abnormal electrical brain discharges and brain waves,[10] a reduced volume of the brain's left hemisphere,[11] and a reduced size of the primary pathway connecting the brain's two hemispheres.[12] The effects of years of repeated abuse on the brain's stress hormones may cause such changes.[13] The left hippocampus may be particularly vulnerable to traumatic stress,[14] and a smaller left hippocampus and dissociation appear to be related.[15]

Along with changes in the brain, a profound difference in the structure of the mind can result from abuse or neglect. The separate states of mind of infancy, called behavioral states, which would normally integrate over time into a cohesive personality,[16] may not unify.[17] This lack of unification becomes an advantage and is reinforced during the abuse. According to one theory, the advantage is that certain systems of cell connections remain separate. The systems for functioning in daily life are kept apart from systems that are responsible for a person's survival during severe threat.[18] In this way, traumatic experiences are registered and stored separately from the parts of a person's mind who must function and present themselves to the outside world.

Some researchers see DID as the most extreme form of dissociation between systems of daily life and systems of defense and survival.[19] According to this theory, when trauma is most overwhelming and/or prolonged, each of the two categories of systems breaks down within itself and remains separate into adulthood. The system for daily life might break down into single systems such as caretaking (the mother) or exploration (the schoolchild, the worker). The system of defense might include fight (the defender or protector) or hypervigilance (the guard, the perpetually vigilant child). Each identity within the system of defense would take control on cues they learned through traumatic experiences. As Samantha said, Cecelia's cue is "any sexual overtures made towards me," and The Smart One appears for "anything that has to do with a lecture, an assignment, or somebody telling me that there's something I need to learn." Samantha, as a part strictly for daily life, is in control for the tasks she does best.

However, no one fully understands how single systems such as mother, worker, defender are formed, or how these systems evolve into individual parts with their often strong sense of personal identity. Some researchers think that dissociated parts develop identities through accumulated, separated memories. Each accumulation of memories would eventually become an individual but one-sided identity,[20] with her or his own characteristics, behaviors, self-awareness, and purposes determined by that part's particular experiences.[21] Self-hypnosis may also play a role over time in creating each parts' characteristics and in visualizing them.[22] Traumatic experiences must generally be repeated over time for the creation of dissociated identities to take place.[23] However, once the mind has created dissociated identities during childhood and adolescence, a single new trauma in adolescence or a crisis perceived as traumatic during adulthood can cause the creation of a new part of the mind with its own identity and function if the already existing parts are not equipped for that particular role.[24] Evidently some children's minds also create a dissociated identity based on a single traumatic event.[25]

Memories in Fragments, Personality in Fragments

The nature of traumatic memory helps explain how traumatic events are stored as separate groups of memories or memory fragments that can evolve into dissociated identities. Ordinarily, the brain stores experiences in verbal and immediate memory so that a person can think or speak about those experiences. Terrifying, overwhelming, inescapable events called trauma are not stored in words for immediate recall.[26] Of all traumas, childhood abuse seems to result in the most thorough memory blockage from those parts engaged in daily life.[27] Being loved and abused by the same caretaker is perhaps the most difficult trauma of all to assimilate in normal memory[28] and may be the most likely type of trauma to cause dissociation.[29] The child's need for at least part of her mind to preserve the attachment to the abusive caregiver appears to be the reason why memories of abuse by a caregiver are the most difficult for that part of the mind to retrieve.[30]

Instead of being stored in words for immediate retrieval, traumatic memories are stored as nonverbal fragments: emotions, behaviors, smells, images, sounds, or body sensations. These memories belong to the identities in charge of defense and survival.[31] Even when the original danger has long passed, such memory fragments or reminders of such fragments remain cues that the identity with no knowledge of traumatic events must lose conscious awareness and relinquish control of the body to another part of the mind. My interviewees mention a variety of cues, such as "I feel pressured and overwhelmed," "a certain kind of cigarette that my brother used to smoke," "any sexual overtures made towards me," "the theme music to a certain cartoon," "the sound of a zipper unzipping."

Traumatic memories tend to be frozen in time rather than altered by subsequent experiences[32] and can freeze a part's age, making it logical that those parts created through traumatic memories often remain emotionally and cognitively in childhood and adolescence. Years after the trauma has ceased, those parts continue to react to trauma-associated smells, sounds, sights, or sensations just as they did during the actual trauma. Years of repeated explanations and discussions with therapists and with the adult part(s) of the mind engaged in daily life are required for young parts to accept that the world around them has changed, making their original roles redundant, though they may still be useful in other ways.

Years later traumatic memories may return as fragmented, intrusive, and upsetting replays of the event, called flashbacks; in coded form as drawings or nightmares; as physical sensations such as gagging or body pains; or through reenactment of the event through self-abuse or through seeking out abusive sexual, physical, or emotional experiences with others. Younger parts may begin to disclose their memories to the adult part who had been protected from such memories so that a woman then learns why the smell of a certain type of cigarette causes her to suddenly lose consciousness. Samantha has recovered many memories, as she previously described, but only since she began therapy sessions during which other parts began talking to her therapist, sessions Samantha could not remember. However, she still gets a "funny smell" in her nose and is switched to another part of her mind whenever she hears the theme music to a certain cartoon, but she cannot recall what happened as a child whenever that music was played.

THE VERSATILITY OF A MIND SHAPED LIKE SAMANTHA'S

Samantha is a part of her mind who did not register the abuse and store abuse memories and, according to her description, she was the first identity. However, the mind is versatile in its abuse-related structure. For example, a child's first identity may perceive too much of the abuse and temporarily or permanently become unable to function in the outside world.[33] Other parts then interact with the outside world alternately, singly, or in combinations. Often there is one identity, the "host," who primarily controls the body and shows herself to the outside world, but this identity is not necessarily the first one. At times, there is no single host, as Samantha illustrates. Sections of the interview with her revealed that Samantha's daily speech and actions on all practical matters including grocery shopping, cooking, and caring for a sick child reflect three identities: Samantha, The Smart One, and Julia.

An identity's purpose can be as broad as carrying out all intellectual activities, like Samantha's The Smart One, or as narrow as saying no like Samantha's four-year-old part fragment called Marla. While one part may be created for only one mission, then remain dormant, another part may take over the body continuously for weeks, months, or years. The barriers between parts can be impermeable or one-way or two-way permeable,[34] enabling some parts to have extensive and other parts only limited knowledge and contact with the rest of the mind. While one person may have only one other part created from a set of trauma incidents, another person's mind may consist of over a hundred parts or part fragments, with each containing a single traumatic memory.[35] Anywhere from three to thirty identities appear to be the most common.[36]

There is no known age limit to the mind's ability to form a new identity, and two interviewees formed one new identity during a crisis in their late thirties or early forties. Adding a new, separate part in adulthood can be the only way a person knows how to face new challenges and threats. However, the crucial help in survival and functioning begins with dissociated parts in childhood. As Samantha's experiences illustrate, dissociation among parts:

- Prevents those parts who must function in the outside world from being overwhelmed by numerous inescapable, inhumane circumstances

- Preserves functions that abuse would otherwise destroy, such as the ability to feel love and joy or to concentrate and learn

- Enables a part to be unaware of much or all of the unbearable events so that a person can remain alive, grow, and function

- When abusers are also the caregivers on whom a child depends and to whom a child must remain attached for survival, dissociation among parts enables a part of the child's mind to maintain the attachment as though no trauma had occurred

Dissociated parts then become a highly efficient and ingenious way of storing and living with early childhood events that are overwhelming, repeated, and inescapable and are related to traumatic childhood abuse, an association firmly established by research.[37]

Like Samantha's identities, other women's identities were created out of unique experiences so that even though the process of forming dissociated identities may be the same, each woman's experience of having them is different. Hearing voices was one of Samantha's first signs of having other identities, but some women's first signs are silent, such as different handwritings in their journals, a mute protective presence, or simply periods of amnesia. Samantha has an identity for work and four other adult identities, while some women have only children and adolescents within their minds' systems. Subsequent chapters reveal such variations. Nonetheless, Samantha, with her clearly defined identities, some of whom spoke with me, and her insight into them, provides an excellent basic lesson in the necessity, functions, formation, and inner logic of having dissociated identities when repeated, inescapable horrors are part of a child's life.

Points to Keep in Mind

- Having dissociated parts is the mind's protective response to prolonged childhood trauma.

- Each dissociated part has one or more specific roles or functions and may work alone or with other parts to protect against memories and perceived outside threats, or to help with functioning in daily life.

- Dissociated parts created to help a traumatized child can be both a help and a hindrance later in life.

- A child with parts is not likely to question her experiences of hearing voices or feeling that she is outside her body, and later in life may assume they are the norm.

- People with minds in parts can pass as unified personalities even among intimates.

2

Dissociated Identities Inside and Out

[While talking with you] I've had to suppress some urges to say different things [because] I'm trying to stay right in the middle and hold the whole picture. There was a point earlier [during the interview] that if I talked, I would have been talking a lot different. And I think the discussion in my head was like, "You'd better keep your mouth shut or she's going to think you're committable," or "You don't know what bad things might happen" or "You're going to get in trouble." [So] *I'm* doing all the talking here and my goal is to stay forty years old and to converse in a big kind of way. But I also am aware of other parts of me, like it might be a part that doesn't want to talk at all but somebody else is like, "Tell her about this! Tell her about this!"

—*Barbara, a forty-year-old social worker*

◉

Barbara's words illustrate that various parts of her mind in all their diversity were listening and often influencing presences during interview sessions. The same was true of almost all my interviewees.[1] It took me a while to grasp the fact that even when no other parts spoke with me directly, they were listening to every question I asked and, in some cases, were feeding responses to the identity speaking to me. After all, they were there when

37

the abuse occurred and, together with the identity speaking with me, they constitute the memories of the past and present experiences I asked about. Also, most of their lives they protected the identity speaking to me and some, especially the parts who are children, were suspicious of me. Over the years, the women I interviewed told me in speech and writing about the vivid presences inside their minds, what their roles are, and how it feels to have them inside and alternately emerge to take control of the body.

VARIATIONS AMONG IDENTITIES

In the mind's eye of each part, she or he has an identity that differs from all other parts even while, to the onlooker, all of them have one face and body. Parts view themselves as individuals, some of whom differ in gender, race, or religion. They may see the body as not belonging to them or as reflecting their own self-perception so that a seven-year-old male part, for example, will refuse to believe that he inhabits a fully grown female's body. Instead, parts see themselves as looking ideal for their roles, and they behave accordingly. Samantha's descriptions of her parts The Smart One and Cecelia in Chapter 1 are illustrations of such self-perceptions. The Smart One perceives herself as forty-three, tall, thin, liking mauve suits, having an abrupt manner, and being very smart, while Cecelia perceives herself as fourteen, short, with curly red hair, freckles, and liking shopping, flirting, jeans, T-shirts, and going barefoot. In contrast, this is how Samantha describes herself:

> I'm five foot two; overweight—not horribly overweight but over-weight—I have glasses [and] short curly brown hair. . . . I like yellow [clothes]; I'm good with kids—and I think that's about it.

Along with differences in looks are differences in sensation and physiology. Samantha wears glasses while Cecelia does not, possibly because

Samantha (not Cecelia) needs glasses. The same pair of eyes can have two or more ranges of vision, depending on which consciousness controls the brain. Such differences can hold true for the senses of hearing, taste, and touch; for body pains and illnesses, allergies, rashes, heart rates, disabilities, muscular strength, endurance, left- and right-handedness, immune system responses, and responses to alcohol, street drugs, and medications, to mention only some of the physiological uniqueness that characterizes dissociated parts of the mind.[2] These differences can have their own logic, depending as they do on the part's age, experiences, purposes, and emotional state. Parts who have secrets they are afraid to tell may be dumb or able only to whisper. When a certain part is dominant, the body's skin may react to past abuse by breaking out or the muscles by going into a spasm. One part of Reba's mind took her father's brutal physical abuse, and only when that part is in control of the body does Reba stutter and have a severe muscular contraction, affecting her ability to walk and to use her right arm. Eyes and ears of one identity may be closed to all perception because that identity could not bear to see or hear the truth of her experiences. One researcher recounts having had four clients for DID who had been in programs for the deaf because deaf parts of their minds were in control most of the time.[3]

Conversely, an identity may be unusually acute in one or more senses. During her childhood, Barbara's mind created a dog identity to help Barbara through the repeated humiliation of having to suck her father's penis. As a dog offered a "bone" Barbara changed the context from ordeal to treat. When Barbara is in her Dog Girl state of consciousness she has a heightened sense of smell and hearing. With such striking differences in identities' self-perceptions, it is understandable that the truth of sharing one body can be very difficult to accept.[4]

Each part has likes and dislikes that can cause amusing dilemmas in choosing what to wear in the morning, prompting some women to select their clothing the night before so that internal quarrels will not make them late for work. When I asked Barbara in what way her clothing dilemma differed from ordinary indecisiveness, she replied,

Say I'm me and I go to the closet and I know I want to wear black so I pull out black. Then there's a shift in my consciousness, in my sense of who I am, and all of a sudden I'm this flamboyant self who only wants to wear the most bright, gaudy thing in the closet. And she'll take that out, and then somebody [else] is like, "No no no, don't make me wear that!" And so I kind of go through a little battle. I guess it's subtle. To somebody watching me they might think that it's like you were saying, "Hmm, I'm sort of inclined to wear this, but I'm sort of inclined to wear that." But it's not like a "sort of," it's adamant from each part of me; it's like, "No way! I'm not going to be caught dead in that!"

Barbara was once halfway through her long commute to work when she noticed that she was wearing a baggy sweater, torn jeans, and sneakers, hardly appropriate attire for a social worker on the job.

Grocery shopping can be equally perplexing when a woman enters a grocery store to buy practical items and finds herself at the cash register with a cart full of cookies, candy, and play-dough.

Differences in food preferences can be confusing to partners and friends who do not understand why a woman is decisive about drinking her coffee black or detesting fish one day and a day or a week later she adds cream to her coffee or suggests a seafood restaurant for an evening out. The quantity as well as quality of her food may differ depending on the requirements of her parts. Several women told me of parts who eat only certain foods or are anorexic or bulimic. These potentially dangerous differences are often related to oral sex during childhood, the seeking of emotional soothing through food, or the urge to be fat as a protection against men. Only Samantha and her four-year-old part Marla can eat, for example, and Marla eats only ice cream. Samantha told me that she does not know why the other parts of her mind refuse to eat, but she does know that eating makes them throw up. However, when I asked Samantha why Marla eats only ice cream, she inadvertently gave a possible reason why most of her other identities regurgitate anything put in the mouth:

At the beginning [when I was about four], Marla only ate ice cream because when my father would stick himself in our mouth, we would throw up. And then he said, "Okay, if you can do it without throwing up, I'll get you some ice cream." And Marla said, "Okay, I like ice cream; I'll try." And she tried and she did it. And so she got the ice cream. So every Sunday night he would take Marla out for Rocky Road ice cream. But no one else could eat because eating made them throw up.

Other parts also have talents and hobbies that differ as widely as those among individuals in the outside world. A woman may be able to read music, play an instrument, draw, paint, do woodworking, ride a horse, or cook special dishes in one identity but not in others. Only one of her identities may be able to drive a car, repair electrical appliances, speak a foreign language, or solve mathematical problems. Some of these talents may have been relegated to a part of the mind free from knowledge of the abuse in order to enable the talents to develop and to preserve them. Such variations can make a person unusually versatile and accomplished but also dependent on having the appropriate part take control at the right time.

With such individuality, it seems logical that dissociated identities often have first names and some have middle and last names as well. I originally assumed that the earliest identity named other parts of her mind, just as parents name their children. Although sometimes one part of the mind does name other parts, many of my interviewees' parts seem to have been created with names and to have always known their own names. By age seven, Reba already knew one of her other parts' names because she would hand in school papers signed "Kelly Marie." Reba could not explain to her puzzled teacher why she put that name on her papers and said simply, "Because that's the name it's supposed to be." Other women have first learned their parts' names as adults, when the voices they had heard for years finally introduced themselves as identities with names. When I asked Gabbi how she knew her other parts' names she said, "How do I know your name or my friends' names—they just exist, like anybody else."[5]

Some parts' names have their own logic, often related to the abuse or to the part's particular function, age, or place of "birth." A part of Ellie's mind carries the name of her beloved grandmother, in whose formerly safe house Ellie's father once raped her. Ellie's other parts' names have no such direct associations. Gabbi's one male part has her abusive brother's middle name, but Gabbi is not sure why, and her female parts simply carry unrelated women's names. Barbara's parts called GaGa and Slugger were both named by one of her other parts. GaGa received her name because she is an infant part and cannot speak, and Slugger because he is a tough and mean part of Barbara's mind. Elizabeth's Nurse Nancy takes care of all friends' and relatives' injuries and has done so since Elizabeth was a child; Reba's Twelve and Sixteen were created at those ages; and Caroline's Montana Girl appeared when Caroline moved there as a child.

Because multiple parts alternate control of the body, sleep requirements may be quite different from the usual eight consecutive hours. Some women who have parts are able to work exceptionally long hours without any break for sustenance or rest. Barbara, Lucy, Elizabeth, and Ruth explicitly attribute their ability to override fatigue to their parts.[6] This ability may be partly due to the fact that at least some parts are able to sleep while one or more others are awake. Elizabeth is certain that throughout childhood at least part of her mind never slept. She later learned that part's name, Night Guard, who remained vigilant to catch the first sounds of her drunken father's nighttime return home and ascent to her bedroom. As an adult, she used to have lucid dreams, half awake, half asleep. Samantha's part The Smart One said that when she is not needed she can sleep if she wishes. Samantha explained in Chapter 1 that when she had a paper to write for school but was so tired she had to sleep, she would suddenly find it was four in the morning and her paper was typed. Thanks to The Smart One, Samantha's system was reinvigorated so that part of Samantha's mind, otherwise exhausted by her father's nightly demands, could succeed in school. This theme was echoed by Ruth, a physician, who told me that her part called The Physician does the medical work. The Physician is able to sleep even while Ruth stays out half the night. The Physician's mind "shuts down," Ruth says. Ruth awakens exhausted the next morning but feels refreshed the minute she enters her office and The Physician takes over.

Being able to separate from fatigue can have drawbacks, as Barbara and Elizabeth have found. This is especially true when parts, who often do not perceive the body as belonging to them, disregard the body's needs for sustenance and rest. Barbara appears to have parts who do not sleep. When she is tired, she can easily separate from tiredness: "[Y]ou just shut that tired part away and go to someone who doesn't sleep." Elizabeth would think all night long and sometimes felt like she had not slept for a year. Eventually, for both women, complete physical exhaustion or even illness were signs that their bodies have limits and needs that no part should ignore.

Parts' Typical Functions

Unique as they are, parts do tend to fall into two overarching categories divided by age. First, there are child and adolescent parts, most of whom are frozen in time. Whether passively existing inside the body or taking active control of it, only the past is real to most of these young parts of the mind. Naturally, they consider the dangers of the past still present and their original functions still necessary. Those child parts who are aware of the present nonetheless remain emotionally and intellectually children trying to fulfill their original functions in spite of their changed circumstances.[7] Although these parts appear obviously out of character once the body reaches adulthood, they blended indistinguishably during childhood.[8] Second, there are adult parts who have aged along with or are older than the body. They generally perform an adult's tasks such as provide soothing and wisdom or go to work.

All parts tend to have roles or job categories related to the trauma in their lives, and those roles help explain their attributes. Researchers have categorized dissociated identities in various ways, sometimes by gender or age group, for example, but also by job categories.[9] The following categories

are ones I have found most frequently among my interviewees' identities
and the ones I consider most useful in understanding my interviewees' life
experiences.

Self-Presentation

Among all other parts of the mind reside one or more who most frequently
present themselves to the outside world. The *host* is the term I use for such
a part. The host is the part who controls the body most of the time during
a given time period. This period can be weeks, months, years, or a lifetime. "The host," "the outside person," or "the presenter" are the terms
Veronica used to describe the part shown to the public. Barbara referred to
such a part when she said, "There's a sense of me as in who's the most common person that people meet when they meet me." The host is not necessarily the body's original identity and may or may not be one single part.
Some women have a host made up of several parts who pass as one. Such
a host may be the identity present from earliest childhood, an identity
formed later, a combination of the two, or a combination of later identities. Samantha illustrated in Chapter 1 how multiple parts can together be
the host.

Sometimes other parts describe the earliest identity as having been "put
to sleep" because she could not bear the abuse. If a woman can process her
traumatic past, the earliest identity may feel safe enough to emerge once
again. Reba, for example, "went deep inside" when she was five and did not
come out again until therapy during and after college when she joined with
another part and became what Reba calls the current "host" or "main person." On the other hand, Caroline does not know whether or not she is her
body's earliest identity or whether she came later, something she hopes to
ascertain through therapy. Samantha knows that she was the earliest
identity and that she was born forty-three years ago. However, for reasons
unknown to her, Samantha considers herself to be sixteen years old, the age
at which she became engaged to her first husband and her father stopped

abusing her. Samantha's self-perceived youth may be one of the reasons why The Smart One and Julia, both forty-three, are indispensable as cohosts.

I soon learned the difficulty of asking an interviewee whether or not she is her body's earliest identity. A brief excerpt from my interview with Samantha is an example. Samantha had been telling me about each of the other parts and why they came. She had told me that four identities were alternately in charge most of the time and had already spoken of The Smart One, Julia, and Cecelia.

Q. Wasn't there a fourth?
A. And there was me.

Q. You were first?
A. Right.

Q. Is the question appropriate why you came?
A. I think I was just born. [We both chuckle.]

This interview excerpt illustrates the distinction I had made in my own mind between the earliest identity and later ones, in contrast to Samantha's reference to herself as simply a fourth identity on a par with The Smart One, Julia, and Cecelia. In a similarly awkward fashion, I once asked Ellie if she, the identity I was interviewing, was the same identity who generally presented herself to the world. Her appropriately humorous reply was, "[You mean,] am I the real me?" [We both laugh.] Ellie did not directly answer my question but stated that although some of "the others" blend very well with her, most are distinctly different.

Because of a possible variety of hosts and other parts, a woman's range of character traits may be unusually wide and sometimes conflicting. Nonetheless, the parts were able to pass as one in childhood and generally continue to do so in adulthood, despite the occasional awkward situation. Hosts help with the indispensable task of passing as "normal."

Sex

Incestual sexual abuse had been part of all my interviewees' childhoods, and all had one or more identities who took the sexual abuse. Judging by the women I interviewed, some parts who took the abuse are children, but those who took the abuse and are sexually active over time are adolescents. Although an adolescent victim is shockingly young from an adult's perspective, to a child, adolescents appear mature and savvy, with bodies markedly changed and ready for sex. Thus, it is logical for the abused child's mind to create an adolescent part for sex, a part whose voice, later in life, can pass as an adult's.

Some sex-specific parts have women's names, like Gabbi's Heather, or job-specific names, such as Samantha's The One Who Performs the Sexual Functions, as Cecelia used to be called.[10] Evocative or derogatory names are also used, like Black Betty, Slut Girl, and Bitch, depending on how the other parts, including the host, perceive the sexual part. Some sex-related parts seem similar to Samantha's Cecelia, sharing her necessary trait of liking sex with any man. Barbara's sixteen-year-old, black-haired Slut Girl is a good example, as Barbara, who calls her parts "ways," explains:

> I used to have Slut Girl [but not] until I was a teenager. Slut Girl [would] take control at times during sex, especially if there were younger ways in me who were scared and who might possibly create problems. She also came out and took control during sexual abuse where sex was being forced and there was nothing to prevent the powerlessness except to pretend it was my *choice* to be sexual.

Cecelia and Slut Girl, both adolescents, changed the context of abuse into pleasant, or at least tolerable, sexual experiences. Gabbi's Heather, also an adolescent, specifically seeks abusive sex, perhaps partly because that is the only kind she knows, and because her body learned to associate pain with sexual arousal.[11]

Ellie's sexual torture brought forth a male part based on a different type of logic. Ellie tells about a gender transformation in response to torture:

> Julie Ann couldn't handle what was going on so she turned into a boy, Jimmy, 'cause boys can handle stuff like that. Not only that, there was a lot of sexual torture, and I suppose . . . I must have felt that what was happening to me was because I was a girl, and if I wasn't a girl and didn't have any place for them to stick those knives, they wouldn't do it. So I just became Jimmy; I was a boy! And Jimmy has kept that part of the pain.

Reba's parts Jo and Andi and Barbara's part OwOw are neither male nor female, an attribute possibly based on a protective logic similar to Ellie's.

Ellie has nine parts and Reba once had forty-two who took the sexual abuse and torture. None of them changed the context into tolerable situations. Their roles were to take the abuse whether they liked it or not so that Ellie's part Joy Lee and Reba's parts Beckilynn and Angel could be "good girls," maintain an image of living in a happy family, and function at home and at school. Ellie and Reba were both abused by numerous relatives and strangers, all pedophiles who enjoyed practicing live sadistic pornography in groups, sometimes in ritualistic settings. Possibly the sheer number of abusers contributed to the number of sex-related parts and to the improbability of creating any single part who could change the context into something positive or bearable.

Concentration and Learning

Safeguarding the ability to learn at school and concentrate on the job is an essential function and frequently found among dissociated identities.[12] Some identities take on concentration and learning as their particular roles. All other identities may contribute to the effort by protecting other parts, including the host, from feeling or knowing about the abuse so that the protected parts can concentrate and process information. These parts protect the person from academic failures and from being considered "learning disabled," often the fate of traumatized children.[13] Seven of the eight women who participated in this study were not consciously present at school at least part of the time, and the eighth, Lucy, suspects that another part took the tests although the Lucy part was conscious in class. Two interviewees know that they had parts who consistently performed schoolwork, and three have parts specifically responsible for the workplace. Barbara's Working Girl, Samantha's The Smart One, and Caroline's Working Woman are characterized by the absence of emotion, and among the three, only The Smart One cares about or is responsible for anything other than her profession. With their one-track minds, they can be an employer's dream.

Protection

What does a child in an abusive household need most? As expected, parts who try to take action to protect the host from harm appear to be quite common among people who have dissociated identities.[14] Protector parts come in many varieties, but often they are male, have the courage to occasionally fight back at abusive adults, and discourage behavior that they perceive as dangerous. Women can find themselves unusually physically powerful when a protector part controls the body.

Barbara describes her male part Slugger as looking like a tough teenager and sounding "loud and mean," like her abusive father and older brother, people with the power she herself so badly needed. Slugger sees his persecutors as models of strength and power and imitates them accordingly. Other women's protectors may adopt their looks, speech, and behavior from images of the macho male seen in television and advertising. Although such images may be extreme to the point of caricature, they are hardly too extreme for the circumstances that brought them forth.

Barbara is somewhat fearful of Slugger and told me that a sure way of keeping him at bay is to wear a dress. Slugger, true to his tough-guy role, "would hate to wear a dress."[15] Protectors who are tall, muscular, and perhaps armed men are evidently frequent[16] but not all protectors necessarily look the part. For example, Reba's female part of the mind called Circle had the courage to fight back at Reba's parents and now carries on that role against other aggressive people in Reba's life. Even Samantha's four-year-old part Marla is a would-be protector. As a part created solely to say no to Samantha's father, she is pitiful evidence of a child's insoluble dilemma in having to defend herself against a parent she loves and on whom she is dependent.

Nurturing and Wisdom

Lacking parents who can be reasonable and wise, some abused children create their own. At times, such parts are perceived as older than the host and motherly looking. Ellie's part called Edna is older than Ellie and ages with her so that she remains older. Edna mothered Ellie as a child, providing nurturing, strength, and a calming influence for all other parts of Ellie's mind. Elizabeth once had several mothers inside her, not all of them good ones. One, however, was called The Good Mother and during Elizabeth's childhood tried to live up to her name for Elizabeth, as the host, and for Elizabeth's child parts. Over time, The Good Mother learned how to internally defend Elizabeth just as Elizabeth now defends her two daughters. Reba's part called Circle, a defender, also serves Reba with wisdom and looks her part: "Circle considers herself Native American, and that's what she looks like, very wise," Reba said. "She's an adult, [but] I don't think she has a definite age." Circle "watches over" all other parts of Reba's mind, sometimes taking over at the end of the workday to make sure that the tired Reba eats and gets to bed at a reasonable hour so she can get up early for the next workday.

Organization

With many dissociated parts running one body, some degree of internal organization is essential for smooth functioning. One researcher mentions parts for organization as among the most frequent types of dissociated parts, calling them "administrators" and classing them as having the dual role of wage-earning and organization.[17] Two published personal accounts tell of a part who is "historian" or "librarian" and record keeper.[18] Along these lines, Samantha, Elizabeth, and Reba have parts solely for the purpose of organization and/or memory, although their specific activities may differ.

Samantha's part called The Organizer came when Samantha was eight. That was the age at which her father's "punishments" increased and several new identities were created, and a time when a more organized internal structure was necessary for Samantha's functioning. The Organizer switches different parts into control as the occasion demands. Furthermore, she swiftly relays information to other parts of Samantha's mind just before they are switched out so that they will know the context of the situation they are about to enter. Samantha explains,

> If I'm coming back because one of the kids has just asked me to make them some soup [and] all of a sudden I'm there and the kid's staring at me and I don't know what was going on, that's real awkward. So it's easier if The Organizer just tells you, "Anne just asked you for a bowl of soup." It's hard to be dropped in the middle of a scene and not know what's been going on.

Part of The Organizer's ability stems from the fact that she knows and can remember what has happened, maintaining a steady short-term memory. With true organizational flair, The Organizer also "keeps records" in a filing cabinet from which she can retrieve Samantha's long-term memories. A part who maintains continuous awareness and who holds a person's life history in memory appears to be common among people who have dissociated identities.[19]

Elizabeth's organizing identity is a female called The Umbrella, and Elizabeth thinks of her as the "cruise director." Elizabeth was sometimes able to hear The Umbrella giving instructions to other parts to get Elizabeth through the school day, "You take the test; you do math; you do this; you do that." As Elizabeth says, "I didn't even have to pay attention because I knew she would take care of things." Reba's part called The Helper is "kind of a grandma," Reba says. "She's an older woman [and she] wears her hair in a soft bun." Before therapy, The Helper coordinated and controlled the forty-two child or adolescent parts of Reba's mind so that Reba, as the host and adult professional, would neither be disabled by internal chaos nor confronted with child abuse memories before she was ready. During therapy, The Helper choreographed child parts' forward movements into Reba's consciousness so that Reba met only one or two younger parts at a time. In this way, Reba was able to work through each dissociated abuse memory without being overwhelmed. Reba gratefully attributes her ability to function throughout life to The Helper.

Pain

A child's inescapable pain during emotional abuse, rape, beatings, and torture is a major factor in the need for psychological and physical numbness. A specific part will sometimes take whole abuse experiences, including the physical pain, although taking the whole experience can eventually become too much for one part. In that case, either a different (perhaps older or male) part is created for the experience, or aspects of the abuse are distributed among parts so that pain, for example, goes to a part created to take pain. Two women told me of parts whose jobs are solely to take pain. From the ages of six to nine, Reba had a part called It who was inanimate and therefore could take torture without feeling it. It split off from a part called Kelly Marie in order to help her endure the abuse. In contrast, Samantha's The One Who Feels the Pain is an eight-year-old female part who can feel but who is paralyzed. Her paralysis has a logic: "she wasn't able to try to get away from the pain," Samantha said. The One Who Feels the Pain's job is to take all pain, physical and emotional, but her face never shows it because another part of Samantha's mind, the eight-year-old female Whipping Boy, is also present for pain and shows no expression. Thus, the immobile, blank-faced child perfectly served her father and avoided intensification of the abuse that any negative reaction would have caused. Only Samantha and The One Who Feels the Pain get sick, while all other parts of her mind remain well. Headaches and childbirth are the only pains Samantha has always been able to feel and remember.

Self-Injury

The majority of my interviewees have repeatedly cut, hit, or burned themselves or injured themselves by other means. Their experiences concur with other studies showing that self-injury occurs among 30 to 40 percent of people who have DID or other forms of dissociation.[20] Self-injury provides temporary release from overwhelming emotions, sensations, and other experiences related to the effects of trauma when verbal release is impossible or insufficient. Specific parts sometimes carry out the injury, wishing either to injure themselves, another part, or the body. Gabbi's part called Casey is a female about whom Gabbi knows little except that she is unruly, suicidal, drives fast, and cuts the body. My interviewees Barbara and Samantha each have one male part who sometimes cuts the body. Barbara's Slugger is rageful and has violent wishes, but when he injures the body, he means to protect Barbara by preventing her from acting in a way that could once have risked abuse. Slugger illustrates that parts who injure the body can be protectors whose strategies are harmful. Barbara also has other parts who came out during certain events and who cut in various ways and for various reasons: to gain control, express anger, prove courage and ability to endure pain, feel in touch with the body rather than "floating off in space," and simply to see blood. Elizabeth has two unnamed parts who used to take over the body to cut and burn it, then depart, leaving Elizabeth to find herself wounded. Because self-injury serves many trauma-related purposes, the job categories of self-injurious parts are manifold and can vary from suicide prevention to the prevention of revealing secrets.

Containment and Preservation

My interviewees also mentioned functions that tend to fall under the job category "keeper of . . ." such as parts who keep or contain the memory of a single abuse episode or keep a single, basic function such as eating or defecating. For example, Samantha has a three-year-old part whose sole job is to use the toilet. Another part can keep the feeling of rage in general, or the feelings of hate or love for an abusive parent or other person. Such parts, or part fragments, can have only that function or also fulfill other functions. Samantha and Reba have parts who hold the grief for the unborn children they were forced to abort when impregnated by their fathers. Elizabeth and Caroline each spoke of a part who was keeper of the final way out. This part's function was to offer death as a choice. Yet, Elizabeth emphasizes that having this part was not the same as being suicidal, and Caroline states that her death part was not involved in depression. Instead, the death parts were the means of a final escape; the only way to make things stop forever. Reba's written description of her parts includes a five-year-old called Corrie who was "trained to injure/kill the body" if she revealed the abuse. Corrie once tried to stop the abuse by killing the body. She cut open the left wrist but "it didn't work," Reba wrote. As with Elizabeth's child part, Corrie does not grasp the finality of death but simply wants to do away with "the body" so that it can no longer be abused. Convinced that she has a separate body of her own, Corrie does not realize that if she killed the body, she herself would die.

Keepers can hold states of mind considered too painful for the host or hold emotional numbness, although the host may also feel numb at times. Keepers also preserve the positive in life, such as happiness and pleasure. This ability to feel joy is in striking contrast to the more pervasive emotional numbness of child abuse victims who do not develop dissociated identities.[21] Parts can retain positive feelings and attributes by taking over an emotion or talent to preserve it, or they may protect the host sufficiently so that she can experience and maintain such positives. Samantha illustrated in Chapter 1 how The Smart One preserved Samantha's intellect in the face of parents whose intellectual demands were grotesquely inappropriate to the child's age and who responded to mistakes with torture. Further chapters will bring many more examples of DID as preserver of the positive.

THE EXPERIENCE OF FEELING AND HEARING OTHER PARTS

I would have an awareness that something had gone on, but I could separate from it. If during the day I saw evidence of something that happened last night, like if I had a bruise or I was in a lot of pain [or] was bleeding and I didn't remember how that happened, it would occur to me, "Something happened last night." And it seemed like it happened to somebody else, but it must have been my body because I'm having the effects of it. So I put it together that . . . things happened to The Night Girl and they didn't happen to The Day Girl: . . . "She is kind of me, and I'm kind of her; we are sharing a body—we're different . . ." I guess I couldn't make a whole lot of sense of it. But that was just my *life*; I didn't know how to think anything different, so I didn't question it a lot.

—*Barbara, a forty-year-old social worker*

From my interviewees I tried to learn how it feels inside to have other parts of the mind with their own identities, and to have them long before one realizes what they are. While my interviewees' first experiences of having other identities varied in small ways, two experiences were common to all.

First, they discovered that blocks of time were missing from their memories. Periodic amnesia might sound like an obvious warning signal that something is wrong. Yet, these memory gaps are not dramatic occurrences, like blackouts, but quiet, quick shifts not physically noticed unless they are brought to a person's attention: a clock that just read 10:30 now reads 3:15; a calendar indicates recent days one cannot remember; a friend comments about experiences one should remember but cannot. For example, Ellie told me:

> When I was in high school, a couple of people who I used to hang around with would say things that I had done or said and I had no recollection of it. At the time, I thought they were just trying to make me feel like I was crazy or that I was forgetful—that they were teasing me. And looking back on it now, knowing what I know, it's very likely that I must have done some of those things that they talked about.

A child is not yet capable of puzzling over memory differences, and an adolescent may simply notice that she has a bad memory and instinctively try to hide it. Noticing that she is different from her peers and needing to hide that difference is already an isolating experience for the child. Secrecy and isolation are themes that repeat themselves throughout many of these women's accounts of their lives, both before and after a diagnosis of DID. However, Gabbi was the only woman I talked with who, already in adolescence, suspected something seriously wrong. All other interviewees were adults, often already in therapy, before noticing how much of their lives had not been recorded in verbal memory. We often do not notice the absence of missing objects until we need them; similarly, large chunks of missing time can go unnoticed unless we have reason to look for them. Caroline did not realize until her forties, when her therapist began asking about her past, that entire years of childhood, then later young adulthood, were missing from her memory.

All my interviewees have parts that spoke and/or wrote to each other and often to the host during their earliest years. Hearing voices was, indeed, the second experience common to all my interviewees, though other parts of Gabbi's mind wrote in her journal to Gabbi, as the adult host, and to each other for years before they became audible as voices. One can better understand the phenomenon of such voices by seeing them as the end of a continuum of control over thinking. The continuum would have commonplace thoughts at one end, intrusive, unwanted thoughts in the middle, and uncontrollable voices at the extreme end. A quote by Elizabeth clarifies the difference between the two ends of this continuum. Elizabeth begins by illustrating how the relatively active, controlled experience of thinking about errands to be run shifts to the helpless passivity of overhearing independent voices inside her head.

> I was driving the car, thinking of a few things I needed to do on the way home: I needed to stop at the cleaners, drop off something. But all of a sudden I was like, "Oh!" and I could hear this argument going on in my head. And it was two parts with two other parts, all in this conversation, but two arguing. So now I'm the once-removed person, viewing this conversation in my mind—and it freaks me sometimes when I catch that. And I remember saying, "What's going on?" and one of the parts talking to me about it.

Though these conversations may seem obviously unusual to those who do not experience them, a person who has had them all her life has scant opportunity to realize her difference, so little do we know about what goes on in others' heads. "I didn't know that I was any different from anybody else"; "I thought everybody had that," are comments describing all my interviewees' early years of hearing voices. They know no other way of being and may have no basis of comparison until much later in life, if ever. Their responses correspond with other research showing that children tend to be unaware that their lapses of memory or inner voices are unusual,[22] and that the majority of adults eventually diagnosed as having dissociated identities are unaware of the existence of their parts.[23] My interviewees' experiences further illustrate that the isolation of the mind can successfully keep us in lifelong ignorance of our differences in inner functioning. Only Gabbi and Reba suspected as early as their college years that the conversations and arguments they heard when alone were not common to all. Nonetheless, even as children my interviewees instinctively hid their dissociative experiences from others.

Individual parts can sprinkle traces of their presence for the unsuspecting host in numerous other ways: signing a different name to school papers, wearing clothing the host did not choose, making the hands do or the voice say what the host had not intended, or leaking feelings so that the host suddenly becomes panicked or depressed for no apparent reason. Some women also describe an indefinable sense of the presence of parts even when the parts are quiescent or an inexplicable sense of two lives being lived simultaneously, as further chapters will illustrate.

"All of a Sudden, You'd Just Be Gone"

Usually it was a smooth transition. We really had no clue; it was just automatic: Pam was there and we didn't remember anything. There were a few times when there was panic because we didn't think she was coming, and we were kind of stuck; that was terrifying. But basically it was just a smooth switch that you wouldn't know. All of a sudden, you'd just be gone.

—*Caroline, a fifty-seven-year-old accountant*

Being switched from one identity to another is a crucial part of everyday life for many women who have parts[24] and one that is difficult to grasp. Switching influences how a person speaks and behaves, how she sees herself and the world, what she wishes to do and is capable of doing, and what she experiences and remembers. Trying to understand how the process of switching feels to the person having the experience, I prefaced a few of my questions with "If I were in your head, what would I feel?" the type of question Caroline was answering in the preceding quote when she described being switched to a part called Pam. In their responses, my interviewees described several types of shifts from one part of the mind to another, a process called *switching*.

"It Probably Sounds Like Gibberish"

Perhaps the most rapid type of switch occurs when two or more parts try to speak or act simultaneously. Conflicting gestures indicate that one part wants to take an action another does not. Samantha once experienced such rapid consecutive switches during a desperate battle with a homicidal part for control of the body. Sentence fragments that sound to the listener like gibberish result when several agitated parts simultaneously try to be heard through one mouth. Ellie, who calls her parts "alters," had such an experience at a doctor's office during an examination terrifyingly reminiscent of childhood:

> [The little ones] have been there when a [gynecological] exam has been going on, and things have happened that weren't very pleasant. It probably sounds like gibberish because there are two or three of them that are talking—if you can imagine three voices coming out of one mouth at the same time. The little pieces of it that do make sense have to do with abuse that happened to them. One was screaming at my grandfather, "Don't kill the baby!" One had to do with "Yucky taste; don't like blood." The doctor didn't know what to do. The nurse got more help, and two other doctors and a couple of nurses came in. They held me down—that was the wrong thing [to do]. Eventually I couldn't scream anymore. I stopped and the little ones went away. But it wasn't me that came back; it was an older part who was able to handle that.

Ellie perceives the "gibberish" that came out of her mouth as several parts simultaneously in control of speech, although some observations sug-

gest that rapid switching rather than simultaneous control is more proba-
ble.[25] Only Ellie and Samantha mentioned one such episode each, and both
episodes occurred during a crisis. Such inner explosions may be unusual
because they cause bizarre behavior obvious to an observer and therefore
thwart all attempts to pass as "normal."

"Standing Behind My Eyes"

Far more common is the experience of co-consciousness: having one part
in control of speech and actions while one or more other parts, often including the host, are watching and listening, but helpless. Ellie describes co-
consciousness as "standing behind my eyes unable to control what's going
on, but I can hear and I know what's happening." Describing such episodes,
several women used the terms "standing behind" or "standing beside" the
eyes or the body.

> There were times when I could be walking down the street on my way
> to or from class, or just going for a walk. And I would get sucked back
> into the background, and it was like I was watching myself walk down
> the street. But I didn't feel like I was in my body, you know, I felt like
> I was somebody else watching my body walk down the street. It was
> really strange.
>
> —*Reba, a thirty-two-year-old nurse*

Samantha describes a similar sensation while a part is at work as a lawyer
in the courtroom. She envisions a box similar to a large, old-fashioned cam-
era with Samantha as "photographer" of her own body. By the time I spoke
with her, Samantha had learned from her therapist why the lawyer in the
courtroom and the eyes watching her are both "me."

> I made this thing at one of the hospitals . . . [I]t showed how things
> worked and how I felt. It was this black box that was big on one end

and went to a peephole on the other end. Inside the box, at the big end, was the judge and the judge's table, and the plaintiff and the defendant's table, and me and the other lawyer. And on the outside of the peephole side was me looking in.

Though helpless to control the body walking down the street or defending a client, Reba and Samantha are conscious, watching and listening as their bodies move and speak, onlookers of their own lives.

When Elizabeth was switched but remained co-conscious, she would sometimes notice her mouth twitch, then hear that her speech had changed in tone, volume, or pronunciation. Over time, she began to be able to recognize parts by their speech characteristics. Elizabeth's state of standing behind or beside herself was constant. For years, Elizabeth's consciousness kept a safe distance from her body. She never used the personal pronoun *my* when referring to the flesh and bones that had suffered and betrayed her during childhood. She says,

> It was the body; it was not connected to me. I wouldn't even look at my body. I could look to put makeup on, but still it wasn't me. It was the body getting made up.

"Being Gone"

In contrast, a full switch in consciousness deprives a person of any knowledge of what "the body" is doing. Women describe this experience in various ways, but most often as subtle and instantaneous. "It feels like a blink or like you had fallen asleep or just daydreamed and then come back a week later," Gabbi says, using the analogy of a gentle but split-second occurrence that belies the time gap it can cause. Barbara, Samantha, Ellie, Reba, Caroline, and Elizabeth concur in their descriptions, using terms like "going away," "being gone," "leaving," or simply describing the occurrence after the fact with the switch not mentioned: "It's just suddenly a few hours later or a few minutes later," Samantha says. Ellie wittily describes a mid-conversation switch during a thwarted attempt at truth-telling,

> When I was in high school, I saw the school psychiatrist. . . . I had
> started to say something about what was happening at home, not a real
> big thing, just alluding to it. And the next thing *I* know I was back in
> my classroom. I didn't finish up the session with her. I don't know what
> came out of that, but I gather from my internal conversations with Joe
> that we did a complete reversal of what I was going to say and started
> talking about fishing trips and stuff like that. Fishing! [We both laugh.]

Switching is not always so subtle and unannounced, however, and the sensation may be noticeable either before or during the switch. Two women used the terms "suction" and "vacuum" to describe such a switch. Elizabeth even imitated the sound of a vortex and said, "If there's a smell, it could just whooo, like a vacuum or a suction almost and bring me out of here." Participants in other studies have spoken of moving down inside the mind or being pulled away or down a tunnel inside.[26] Evidently severe headaches portend a switch in some women.[27] Headaches are the most common physical symptoms of having DID[28] and headaches are the physical problem most common among my interviewees, though none mentioned them as a warning signal for switching.

Reba describes a somewhat longer switching process, though still one probably accomplished in seconds rather than minutes. She would see herself fading or feel herself being sucked back into the background, "and then everything would go black." Reba is also now aware of a part trying to come out even before the switch occurs. She uses the analogy of feeling uneasy, "like something's going to happen," or of sensing the presence of someone approaching from behind: "Sometimes it's just like when somebody walks up beside you, and you can see them out of the corner of your eye before they actually get right up to you." Now that Reba, as the host, and the other parts understand and talk with one another, a switch is sometimes simply announced by younger parts inside, but only in the privacy of home: "It's my turn; I want to play," or in the safety of therapy sessions with Judy, Reba's therapist, when Reba will hear a child's voice saying, "I want to talk to Miss Judy."

During interviews, parts other than the host occasionally spontaneously came out to speak with me. Then, if I needed to ask the host a question, the switch back to the host was made at my request. The same can happen when a therapist or other trusted person requests to speak with a certain part or with the host. On an everyday basis, only a few parts are likely to take full control, while others may exert their influence from within. Stress can cause more frequent switching and perhaps a greater number of parts taking control.[29]

According to one interpretation of the switching process, when an emotion is present but not strong, the part who holds that emotion may remain inside, and the host may feel sad, for example, without knowing why. When a critical level of emotional intensity has been reached, the host loses control of the body to the part who is in charge of experiencing that intense emotion. The switch is necessary if the identity in control of the body before the switch cannot allow herself to feel that emotion so intensely.[30] Therefore, the more flexible and expansive the host can become in her ability to remember and feel the past, the less often she will be required to switch. I was surprised to find that strong positive emotions such as joy or delight can also cause a switch. Some women find it difficult to walk through a toy shop or play with their own or others' children or grandchildren without having a child part come out.

Control over the body, including speech and action, was a component of switching common to all my interviewees.[31] The original purpose of a switch was to protect other parts from full cognizance of abuse, and such protection involved taking control of the body and reacting to the abusive events as the controlling part saw fit. In present-day circumstances, even if the trigger is a joyful one, a full switch involves complete control. A switch also dictates both psychological and physical self-perception so that part of a woman's mind may not only perceive herself as having a different hair color or as being a boy or a man, but actually see those attributes when she looks in the mirror.[32] Barbara told me that when a child part has control of the mind she can become unable to feed or take care of herself in her own home. This psychological helplessness can be accompanied by sensations of physical transformation, such as sitting in the driver's seat of a car and finding that one's legs are too short to reach the pedals.

The Process of "Being Gone." My interviewees' experiences suggest that switching is originally activated by a part of the mind separate from the host's will and not under her control. Reba's use of the passive "I would get sucked back," illustrates that the switching process was happening to her, the host, rather than a change she activated. As discussed in the previous section "Organization," if the mind breaks down into increasing numbers of parts, one part may be in charge of responding to cues and control the switching process for all other parts.

The process itself is somewhat a mystery and researchers disagree on how to explain it. Some use the term "self-hypnosis" to describe the underlying process of switching.[33] Others see hypnosis and dissociation as varying degrees of the same psychological process and think that hypnosis is a term describing controlled and structured dissociation.[34] Two of my interviewees offered their perceptions of this debated process.

Samantha, a lawyer, made the process sound simple and for her, it is. "You just close your eyes and put your head back and relax, and then whatever's supposed to happen is going to happen." At an early age one or more parts of Samantha's mind were switched out according to need, as the part called The Smart One told me. Later, during law school, an inner voice would sometimes instruct Samantha on what to do when another part was needed for a law exam: "I'd hear a voice in my head saying: 'Don't worry about it; just take a deep breath and relax and you won't have to worry about it.' So I did." Samantha was once suddenly switched back into control of her body to find herself in bed with an abusive stranger, a time when the Cecelia part normally would have been in charge of the body. I asked Samantha why she thought she had been switched into control at such an inappropriate time. She replied that she did not know why, but added "maybe I lost my concentration." Samantha's choice of the term "concentration" and her need to "just take a deep breath and relax," show that for her, a combination of relaxation and focus is necessary for achieving and maintaining a dissociated state, a combination that seems important to others as well.[35]

Ruth, a physician, who refers to herself as "the core part," gave me a description of her mind's switching process. Ruth says that switching is more difficult and somewhat uncomfortable now that all parts of her mind are closer to being united. When Ruth, as the host, deliberately switches she has to find the way in her mind to the part she seeks by envisioning the part and retrieving that part's emotions, thoughts, and voice. Ruth calls this "creating a connection the long way around," and says intense concentration is involved. One example was a deliberate switch to a male part called The Boss during a therapy session at the therapist's request.

> Basically, I just make my mind go blank, like [I'm] meditating or in a trance. Either I stare at one spot—it's a hypnotic kind of thing—or I close my eyes. The part takes over my body and I go. I'm very close now; I'm almost at eye level with The Boss so I hear everything that's going on but I'm still one step back from the body; like I'm behind the body. And so The Boss will start banging his legs and be much more masculine appearing, the shoulders widen and he sort of slouches on the chair. Or sometimes he gets up just to make himself seem bigger, taller.

For Ruth, making her mind "go blank" seems to allow the switch. Her "staring at one spot" may describe the same mental process as Samantha's "concentration." Both women may refer to the effort to keep the host's mind free of thought so that another part can have active control.

Ruth's and Samantha's accounts suggest a dual process of giving up and taking over. The host relinquishes control by relaxing and clearing her mind so that another part can become dominant. Ruth told me because she is closer to complete integration, she, as the host ("core part"), can inadvertently resume control by thinking. She said it is now harder to keep other parts "in the mind" and described what can happen if her own mind cannot remain blank. "If my mind starts thinking—my mind, the core part's mind—then I can all of a sudden switch out of the part." In years past, when all parts of Ruth's mind were more separate, such an unintended switch from another part to the host was evidently not so easily possible.

Ruth thinks that the process is probably the same, but quicker when the stimulus to switch comes from outside. She describes the quick switch as ". . . automatic, like a phone line that goes directly to a connection." Almost instantaneous is a time span noted by other researchers[36] and one that fits my interviewees' descriptions. However, a few people evidently take many minutes or even hours to switch.[37] The reports of longer time spans may be referring to a deliberate switch initiated by a therapist's request, such as Ruth previously described. During such an overt switch, rapid eye blinking or rolling the eyes upward, a vacant gaze, immobility, a long pause in breath, or a shudder of the body may reveal the beginning of a switch to a knowledgeable onlooker.

Dissociated parts often seem to know, from childhood onward, that it is expedient to pass as one.[38] It follows that the switch will be done in a way that attracts no attention and that overt changes in identity are rare.[39] Yet in the company of a trusted person who knows about the parts, such as a therapist, a woman does not have to hide them. In such liberty, parts who are noticeably distinct from the host, such as male or child parts, may take control, speaking and behaving markedly differently, like Ruth's male part The Boss. Also, parts who in public can pass as the host may allow themselves the welcome freedom of overt self-expression while with a therapist. They are glad to be "out" and to be allowed to be themselves for a while. As a result, facial muscles and posture may gradually change, voice and speech often differ, and examinations reveal that heart rate and respiratory rhythms often change as well.[40] For these reasons, a therapist can notice visible signs of a switch while the person's partner or best friend does not, especially because a therapist would expect to see such signs.

However, a woman can also switch under her therapist's eyes without her therapist noticing.[41] Such switches are extremely difficult or impossible even for specialists to detect. Subtlety and speed in switching are part of the mind's capacity to protect itself. Switching must be subtle and swift because the dual primary roles of dissociated identities are to shield a child's consciousness from knowledge of abuse and to help her function. Sluggish switching would not shield effectively, and noticeable switching would impede a child's capacity to pass as a single consciousness, causing upheaval and social rejection. My interviewees' accounts confirm that when passing as "normal" is paramount, or when responding to a danger cue, the switching process is swift, smooth, and unnoticeable, protecting them from their abusers and from social ostracism.

Despite outward invisibility, brain imaging techniques can now track changes in brain activity consistent with a switch from one identity to another. Studies using such a technique reveal different blood-flow patterns for different autobiographical memories and therefore for different senses of self within one brain.[42] The brain areas that help regulate a person's reaction to external cues of pain and distress were most affected. When an identity who remembered past traumatic experiences and considered the memories her own heard a script about the trauma, those areas of the brain were activated. They were not activated when an identity who had no memory of the trauma, or did not regard the memory as a personal memory, listened to the same script. In this way, some of the brain activity that governs identity changes is visible, even when the person shows no outward sign of switching.

ADMIRABLE MINDS

In studying women's reports about their parts, I discovered how the mind can weave a tapestry of identities that together tell the story of a woman's life. Yet, the variety of parts' looks, traits, sexes, and ages is not for show or color, but for practicality. The range of parts is necessary to better serve the life and functioning of the person as a whole. Yet, with such variety, the extent to which women with dissociated identities can pass as singletons is astonishing. Every woman I interviewed said that no one suspected multiple identities, not even people she knew well. The mind, it seems, is able to function in pieces even while successfully presenting the illusion of wholeness.

Equally surprising is the fact that identity changes can feel subtle, even unnoticeable, from the inside. Years of repeated time gaps made obvious by clocks, calendars, or other people's remarks are often necessary as the first step in recognizing that one's mind functions differently from the norm. Even then, the meaning of such experiences remains elusive.

Yet, from childhood on these women hid their inner voices and memory gaps whether they consciously thought of them as normal or not. It sufficed to sense that their experiences made them different from their peers. This early, instinctual social protection is shared by other children who have dissociated identities.[43] The requirement to pass as belonging to the norm is evidently inherent to the child and may partly determine the types of some of her identities and the switching process.

My interviewees' experiences also showed me the power one part can have over other parts. An identity deemed unprepared to know about experiences in her past may be blind or deaf, so important is it that she not see or hear a memory another part has saved. She may be able to see and hear but not be able to process information another part of the mind has written down or recorded. Conversely, an identity's senses may be unusually acute or her muscles unusually strong depending on her unique experiences and self-perception.

The women I interviewed have also illustrated a major difference between themselves and "singletons" who have a variety of roles in life and are playful with children, relaxed and sociable with friends, and dignified, serious, or commanding with colleagues and employers. The difference is that through all these changes in behavior, a singleton has a continuation of consciousness, control, and ownership: this is *my* intention, *my* thought, *my* action, *my* emotion, *my* experience, and in future years these will be part of *my* memories. A woman with dissociated identities is sometimes deprived of this continuity. Nonetheless, by adulthood she has a set of character traits, talents, and abilities, perhaps broader than the norm, but recognizable by the host and by her family, friends, and colleagues as her identity. This important fact is true for all of my interviewees, although a diagnosis of DID or the sudden quiescence of all other parts can shake that sense of identity, as discussed in the following chapters.

POINTS TO KEEP IN MIND

- Even at a young age, the mind can be savvy and inventive about the characteristics necessary for parts.

- The mind can create whatever age, sex, and other distinguishing features most appropriate for each part's particular job.

- Dissociated parts can preserve positive emotions and talents so that they are free from the influence of trauma.

- The mind can be made up of a variety of identities yet present itself to the outside world as a single identity, so great is the need to pass as "normal."

- The more flexible and expansive the host can become in her ability to remember and feel the past, the less often she will be required to switch.

3

HOW TWO WOMEN
REALIZED THEY ARE
"DIFFERENT"

◉

In this chapter, Reba, a thirty-two-year-old registered nurse, and Gabbi, a forty-two-year-old director of finance, human resources, and administration, describe in their own words their experiences during their early years. Reba's and Gabbi's accounts are excerpts from the transcripts of taped interviews, which I edited and arranged to form a narrative. Their experiences help illustrate the variety of ways a woman may perceive the dissociated parts of her mind before she understands what they are. Reba and Gabbi both realized as young adults that they were somehow markedly different from their peers, although not all people with parts realize that they are different. However, Reba's and Gabbi's language in these excerpts reveals that even after learning about their condition through therapy, they continue to see the other parts as vivid individuals. Such is the power of dissociation, a power that was necessary to protect part of their minds during childhood and enable them to function.

REBA

Reba usually speaks of herself in the plural, a common practice among women with parts even when they understand their condition. She locates her voices and images as being inside her head. "I had these other people in my head that I could talk to." Even in childhood, Reba perceived her "people" as her friends, understanding that they were there to help her but not understanding what they were or why they were there.

"You've Got to Mind Your Dad"

"Sometimes he would come in our room during the night, sometimes during the day—Dad worked odd hours. We'd get home from school, and he'd be home and almost right away start yelling and screaming at us and wanting us to—do things with him. A lot of times he used physical violence to get us to comply, hitting us with a belt or with his fist. If we were to refuse him he'd beat us up until we submitted. [He'd threaten] that he would hurt our younger sister if we didn't do what he wanted us to do. And so we did everything we could to try and keep him from hurting her. He knew that would work, that we would do what he wanted. And there was always the threat afterward that we'd better never tell anyone or he would kill us. And we believed that he would.

"There were times when I'm sure that the mom knew what was happening 'cause she would walk in on the dad abusing us and she would turn her back and walk out.* And we would beg her to protect us and stop it, and she would just say, 'Well, you've got to mind your dad.' She's still never admitted to any of the abuse.

"[I was impregnated] a few times: twice by the dad and once by an uncle, and we were forced to have an abortion [each] time. There were two

---

*In order to distance herself from her parents, Reba often refers to them as "the mom" or "the dad" rather than using the possessive *my*.

other pregnancies by the dad that ended in miscarriage. We were eighteen when we finally got away; [that was] when I left for college."

"I Had These Other People in My Head"

"I think I've always known that I could talk to and see other people in my head that nobody else could see. My mom and other people used to think that I had imaginary friends. As I got older, I knew that they weren't going away and that it was more than imaginary friends, but I couldn't put a name to it; I didn't understand what it was. I didn't know that I was any different from anybody else; I thought everybody had that.

"In some ways, it was comforting to me because I had these other people in my head that I could talk to and that would help me. [But] there were some times when I thought, 'I'm crazy' 'cause people would tell me that I had done things or said things that I didn't remember doing or saying. And so it was a mixture of feeling like I was not normal and knowing that it was something that was helping me, that the other people that I could hear and see in my head were my friends. There were some that helped me get through school, and some that helped me get through abuse—probably we all worked together on that. And there were ones that when they talked to me [they said] that they were going to keep me safe and help me. Sometimes there were ones that were angry and would try and fight back when I couldn't.

"There were days when I knew that I had gone out to get on the bus to go to school, and then the next thing I knew I was home again. I didn't remember being at school, but somebody was there 'cause I would get back papers that had different names on them, and in parentheses my teacher would write *my* name. [When] I was about seven years old, I would get back papers from teachers that had 'Kelly Marie' written on it. And I remember [my teacher] asking me, 'Why are you putting this name on your paper?' And I couldn't explain it to her. It was just like, 'Well, because that's the name it's supposed to be.' But she accepted it; she didn't get angry. As I got older, from about age fourteen, *I* was the one that was more present in school because that was the only place where I felt safe and where I felt like I could do anything right, or do anything good. [But] when I was in college, there were times when I wouldn't remember having been in class or taking exams. And yet, when I got grades back, I did okay. I think it was mostly on days when I was having a lot of stress other than school itself."

"I Realized I Was Different"

"It wasn't till I got in college that I realized I was different. Roommates would ask me why I sometimes wouldn't answer to my name and why sometimes I acted differently than I did at other times. And there were a couple of my roommates that I got to be friends with, and sometimes on the holidays I would go home with them and see the way their families were. That's when I started realizing my family was *really* different [from] other people's families and *I* was different [from] other people.

"I tried to hide it. I couldn't remember being in class, but in my notebooks I had notes from the class. Whichever part of me was there in class kept good notes, so I was able to read through them and get the general idea. People would ask me questions about things that I had done, or places I had been, or what I had learned in my classes. [I] was just trying to fake my way through, so they wouldn't know that I didn't remember where I had been or what had been said in class.

"And I was still hearing and seeing these other people in my head. Sometimes there were arguments [inside] about what I was and wasn't going to do. There were some [people] that were very angry and always wanting to lash out at other people, and [others] arguing that I couldn't do that; that wasn't safe to do. Sometimes they would talk to me and I would talk back to them. But when my roommates were home, [I tried] to hide that because I started realizing they're not that way. I didn't want them to think I was crazy because I would talk to these other people in my head that they couldn't see. When my roommates were home, it was more kind of a silent conversation. [But] I think sometimes my roommates heard some of my alters speaking, they [just] didn't know why I sounded different. Sometimes my roommates said things about me talking to myself and acting weird.

"When my roommates weren't home, I would talk out loud, back and forth with the others in my head. [If someone had been sitting in the room with me during those discussions, they sometimes would have heard me speaking out loud.] They would have just heard one end of the conversation most of the time. Kind of like if somebody was sitting in the room listening to me talking on the phone, they would just hear my end of the conversation.

"It was in college when I first started getting therapy. There was about a week when I did not sleep more than maybe an hour a night. I was getting physically exhausted, and I couldn't understand why I couldn't sleep. I called a medical doctor because I thought maybe there's something physically wrong. He was the one that suggested therapy; he actually called and made the appointment for me, and called me back and told me when it was and that he was going to follow up and make sure I went. And when I got to the counseling center to check in, he was on the phone with the receptionist, checking to see if I had come. That's what got me into therapy. I don't remember the doctor's name. I wish I did so that I could let him know how much it's helped me. It was like a name was finally put to all the things I was experiencing."

"It's Okay with Me"

"I used to feel like it was ruining my life. I hated it because I had a lot of time I didn't remember, [and] I didn't have control. And [there were] problems with some of the parts that would self-injure and then go back inside and leave *me* to deal with cleaning up the mess and pain from it. [But] once we got into therapy and started understanding what was going on, we came out stronger in the end. We learned how to work together and help each other and get some common goals instead of fighting and arguing.

"Since we've gotten cooperation, it's okay with me; I'm not scared of them or anything. It's kind of comforting in some ways. Most of the time I can [feel their presences]. It's just like I know that they're there and that when I'm not at work, if I just need a break, things are still going to get taken care of. I don't know that I can put into words [how] I know that they're there. I can just sense their presence. And when I'm at work [and] they're in the safe room, I can sense that they're still there, and that Circle is kind of watching over me and making sure that I'm safe at work.* When I do get stressed, she's there to remind me to, 'Take a deep breath' and 'Take one thing at a time.' And when we're at home, I can see them, I can hear them, I can feel them, I can talk to them.

"If it's a nice day we'll go sit outside under the trees to eat lunch. And we talk then, just internally, nothing out loud because it's a public place. I listen to them, and we talk a lot about things that we're doing now and things that we're planning. We can pretty much all hear each other. If someone [doesn't] want to hear the others, then they'll just go off on their own. It's kind of strange that we *can* hear each other but we don't *have* to listen if we're not wanting to or not feeling like we can. [At this moment] as you and I are talking, some of them are kind of listening [and] once in a while they're reminding me of different things [to tell you]."

GABBI

In contrast to Reba, Gabbi speaks of herself in the singular. She describes a painful process of perceiving other identities and of gradually realizing that those identities are part of her. Unlike Reba, Gabbi locates her voices as being outside her head. Gabbi's language reveals her struggle to reconcile what she feels with what she knows. She feels that her parts are sepa-

---

*The "safe room" is a structure created in the mind to keep child parts enclosed and out of harm's way while Reba is at work. Safe rooms and other structures are described in Chapter 4. Circle, introduced in Chapter 2, is a wise, adult part.

rate people: "I'm existing over here, they're existing over there. There's no relationship." Yet she knows that they must be part of her: "I understand that they are part of *me*."

"Then I Would Get Dressed and He Would Drive Me to School"

"My father is a physician. He was a very bright guy, first in his class, and always held that over [my siblings and me]. [My parents] had our IQs tested every year, and it was a big issue, 'You're not smart enough.' So we always knew about scores. My sister was blond, and for some reason my parents always wanted blond, and I had dark hair. So there was this constant overtone of 'You're not smart enough, you're not pretty enough, you're not blond enough.'

"I remember [when] I was six or seven years old, I'd be getting ready for school and my father would call me into his room and both my parents would be there. My mother would basically tell me to do whatever my father wanted me to do, and then she would go off to make breakfast for the kids. And then there'd be probably several hours of—I call it torture. It was sexual abuse, but it wasn't just sexual exploitation. My father was into causing pain, and it was important for him that you not cry and that you don't show that anything hurt. So he was into seeing how much pain he could cause before you would show any emotion or cry—and that would just make him more angry. Throughout the whole thing he would be, 'This doesn't hurt.' Then I would get dressed and he would drive me to school.

"When I came home at night usually things were okay; everybody went their separate ways and went to bed. And then I'd get called into my parents' room, usually really late. At night, my mother would stay. Usually the nighttime ones were more ritualistic for my mother. She was into bodily cleansing, so she'd do enemas and douches and those kinds of things to make sure I was clean and pure. Then she'd sit in a chair in the corner most of the time while my father would abuse me. Then I'd go back to bed. Every couple of days that went on.

"My older brother was not—it's so weird now, you know, you talk about this stuff in degrees. He sexually abused me [for] two or three years, but it lacked the cruelty and torture that my father and my other brother had. It was damaging in its own sense, but compared to all this other stuff, it's nothing.

"I had an abortion when I was fourteen; I don't know if I was pregnant by my brother or by my father, but it was one of the two. My mother knew that I was pregnant and brought me out to the front of the clinic, dropped me off, and said, 'Here's some money; go take care of it,' and came back to pick me up. I think she believed it was my father's [child]. But it was one of those things she was never going to admit."

"I Always Felt Like I Missed Something"

"Probably in my midteens is when I first had an idea that there was something very different in the way I behaved and the way I processed things. I came to know that there were times missing and that there were periods that I didn't remember or people thought that I acted very differently. I always felt like I missed something, that things had gone on, [and] I had jumped over them. Originally, I started thinking that I just wasn't paying enough attention. I would consciously try to pay more attention, [but] it didn't change anything. I thought that I was just skipping over things, you know? I'd be here, and then I'd be here, and then I'd be there, and I didn't understand how that happened. People would say I had done something, and [I had] no idea that I had done it. It was the gaps and the things that were missing; it was the absence of any recollection. At that point I didn't have any co-consciousness or any voices.

"[At] school, there were days missing and blocks of time that I had no recollection. But I knew I had been in school, done homework, taken tests. There were times when I knew I had studied for tests and should have done well and didn't do well—and didn't remember taking tests. I knew I had been places and done things that I absolutely could not remember. [In] grade school, my mother would get reports from the teacher. I remember one woman said something to the effect that it was like dealing with different kids: that I could be very sweet, I could be very obnoxious, and that she didn't quite know how to handle me because she never knew how I was going to react or whether I was going to participate or not. And there were times when I was a really good student and did well, and there were times that I did poorly and couldn't read: like one day I could read and the next day I couldn't. Same thing in math.

"I knew around junior high and high school that I would have years [with] a particular teacher, and I have absolutely no recollection of that teacher. But I would look at report cards and obviously I did: there were the grades. But I would have no clue; I couldn't remember the classroom or anything. And I knew from talking to people [that] other people weren't like that. I had friends that had clear recollections of things.

"There were clothes that I had on that I didn't recognize. I would go to be tested and have all kinds of allergies, and then a few weeks later they would test me again and I would have no allergies. From month to month things changed. It's just impossible to ignore those kinds of things. I sort of felt that there were two lives going on at the same time. And [when] I tried to pay attention to that, it became clearer.

"I also knew around that time that I had two very different handwritings; I'd write some things one way and other things in a tiny print. I wasn't quite sure where that was coming from, but I had a sense that they were things I had written because they made sense and fit in; so I did know that they were sort of mine."

"I Don't Think I Really Wanted to Know"

"Originally, I started thinking that it was probably something like a brain tumor or [I had] something major physically wrong. I went through a period when I was convinced that I was dying. But I don't think I ever had any thoughts about it being psychological. When I survived and was still alive and healthy, I knew it wasn't a brain tumor.

"It started coming together when I was in college. Before that, I had clear parts that would come out that I knew had names, identities, and certain behaviors. But I don't think I started labeling it and understanding what it was till I got to college. I was taking a lot of psychology classes and doing a lot of reading. And I started putting a name to it. Before that, I don't think I ever wanted to give it a lot of thought; I don't think I really wanted to know. Once I didn't die during my junior high years and was healthy, the idea through high school and college that it was something like a mental illness was much scarier to me. There was a lot of mental illness in my mother's family. I could see how those people behaved and how they didn't function very well. And then it started becoming even more clear to me that it was probably something more like a mental illness and I really didn't want to know about it.

"Late college, in my twenties, I had a greater awareness that there were more distinct parts of myself that had different identities, different voices, different thoughts, and that there was some sharing between those [parts]. I don't know that I ever thought it was voices, [and] I would not have said it was internal. I felt like I had more sisters, like there were other entities, people, identities that were external. They didn't seem a part of me; they were separate. On some level, I knew they were connected to me, but at that period I don't think I understood. I would never call them internal voices; it was like having a conversation with somebody outside. Another person was there, another sister, another friend. It sounds so weird to tell because now I know that was not the case.

"I don't remember the conversations being verbal; they were much more—I don't how to describe them. A lot of them were written. I did write incessantly when I was younger: I would have things in all kinds of different handwritings and all kinds of different voices. I would have one conversation on one page and one conversation on another page, as if they were very distinct people."

"How Do You Possibly Explain That to Somebody?"

"I thought I understood it well, and then after [my] first meeting [with you] I left thinking, 'I really don't understand anything about how this works. It doesn't make any sense, and it sounds unbelievable.' But I continue to learn and be amazed because as much as I live this and read [about] this, I find it hard to believe. *I* find it hard to understand, so I can't imagine how anybody else can [understand it], certainly somebody who hasn't been here. I mean, it's incredibly difficult to explain.

"Only [during] the last three or four years [have] I *want[ed]* to understand it, [and] only in the last four years have I had any awareness that I could be hearing a single voice or two people having a conversation outside of my head. [Sometimes I can understand what they're saying and sometimes I can't.] It's clear to me that they're younger, male [and] female. They have different opinions than I have [and they're not trying to tell me anything]. They're having an independent experience that has nothing to do with me. It's like somebody in the next room is having a conversation and you're hearing it. It's not me but [yet] it *has* to be me. How do you possibly explain that to somebody?

"It seems that externally there are discrete kinds of individuals, identities, very separate from me but somehow related. [But] there's no interaction; I'm not having conversations with those people; it's not a back and a forth. I'm existing over here, they're existing over there. There's no relationship, which I know doesn't make sense. . . . But these external things are moving closer and closer. I understand that they are part of *me*, but the only way I can deal with them and accept them [right now] is that they are these separate things. And now they're a little bit closer and they're becoming more and more a part of me. And I guess that's the process."

Points to Keep in Mind

- The earliest perceptions of dissociated parts of the mind can vary and be in opposition to each other:

    - The earliest voices can be written and/or vocal.

    - These voices can be perceived as coming from inside or outside the head.

    - The host can perceive the other parts as part of her and helpful, or as separate from her and uninterested in her.

- A child or adolescent is generally incapable of analyzing her dissociative experiences but capable of realizing that they make her different from her peers.

- The fear of being "crazy" or being perceived as "crazy" is a powerful incentive to keeping oneself and others in ignorance of having a mind in parts.

- Simply recognizing or suspecting that she is different from her peers is reason enough for the host to hide her differences.

4

ORGANIZING PARTS OF THE MIND

I was like a zombie; I was so upset all I could do was cry. And then we had this meeting inside—I mean, this is how we deal with things—and we came up with a different plan: Terry's going to do it! She's taken over; this is going to be her thing to do.

—*Caroline, a fifty-seven-year-old accountant*

◉

Disorder and conflict seem inevitable if a group of unrelated people of diverse ages, sexes, temperaments, interests, and talents have to live together without mutual understanding or common goals. This is an apt analogy for the situation of parts who lack a means of organization and conflict resolution. In the preceding quotation, Caroline describes her parts' means of avoiding internal chaos. They meet, discuss problems, listen to each other, and agree on solutions. To help Caroline out of the upsetting dilemma in this case, all parts identify Terry as the most appropriate part for the task. Similarly, other women told me about their organizational process as well as internal meeting rooms and dwelling places. I noted these topics whenever they arose and began to glimpse a complex inner world of activities, architectural structures, household furnishings, and landscapes that help enable a mind in parts to function.

For a person with such a mind, smooth functioning in the world entails the ability to be switched in public unnoticeably and only when necessary for the host's functioning, to make decisions acceptable to most or all parts,

and to pace the retrieval of traumatic memories. Inner organization can
address one or more of these requirements.

MEETINGS OF THE MIND

In the outside world, when a group of people have plans to devise or decisions to make, ideally they meet and talk. This, I found, is what parts do
who have an organizational process. Barbara, a social worker, refers to such
discussions as a part of her life she takes for granted. She considers it unfair
to make a major decision without consulting all of her parts.

> If you're used to being in a marriage, you're not going to take a vacation
> without consulting your partner. Whereas if you're single, you just do
> it. Let's say I'm going to do something, [discussion] is just part of it. So,
> I'm used to being in this kind of thing. I just take it for what it is.

Parts frequently converse informally among themselves and sometimes
with the host as part of everyday life. Hearing voices converse or argue, or
finding written conversations in different handwritings are, or have been,
experiences common to all my interviewees. In a crisis, however, or when
major decisions must be made, all parts may come together in an orderly
fashion. Samantha, Reba, Caroline, Barbara, and Ruth spoke of special
inner meetings for all parts, or at least for all those parts considered capable of offering an opinion on the matter at hand.

Reba and Samantha described a painstaking democratic process in some
detail. Here Reba, a nurse, tells about the inner conversations she heard and
in which she sometimes participated:

> Sometimes they were about things that were going on at work, or there
> were arguments about what I was going to do. It's like we discussed
> almost everything. Whenever there was a decision that had to be made,

especially something important, it was not just *one* that could make the decision. There was kind of like a council, [and] we had to all discuss it and argue over it and come up with an agreement.

Reba's description reveals a democratic council that meets to avoid autocracy of any single part and ensures agreement, which is so essential to smooth functioning.

Agreements, it seems, can be as hard to reach within one person's mind as they are among many people. Like Reba, Ruth, a physician, has an inner democracy and inner arguments. Ruth's arguments seem to lead eventually to reluctant agreements.

> My therapist wanted me to check in with my parts. [All the parts] would get in a circle, and each would tell me what was going on with them for that day, or if there was an issue at hand they would comment on it. Sometimes we would take a vote if I had to make a decision and that was always hard: try to take twenty parts and take a vote on something and it's always ten to ten or fifteen to five; you know, it was never unanimous. And I always had trouble making decisions. I always had—in a regular person it would be ambivalence; in me it was an argument between parts: "No, we shouldn't do that; yes, we should do that."

Similarly, the inner democracy of Samantha's parts is highly organized. A key figure in Samantha's organization is The Organizer. Samantha, a lawyer, describes her organizational structure:

Q. *Are there any other ways you feel your parts?*
A. I can feel them influencing what I'm thinking, like I'll be trying to think about something and my head will keep switching to thinking about something else. Or I'll be doing something and they'll call a meeting, and I'll have to go to the meeting even though I'm doing something. We have somebody who doesn't have a vote. Her name is No One, and she stays out and kind of manages things while we're at the meeting. But

those meetings have to be quick if No One is out 'cause she can't do a whole lot; she's only eight. So we try to make those meetings really quick.

Q. *Now, what might the meeting be about?*
A. Anything really important, like if we're about to do something wrong; like if Cecelia's about to go and meet somebody she met on the Internet. It used to be if we were about to buy something that cost too much—anything that we might be doing that is going to cause problems we have a meeting about.

Q. *And what happens at the meeting?*
A. We talk about what's going on, and then we each vote on what we think we should do. If there's a tie, The Organizer votes and she breaks the tie—she's kind of like the vice president.

Q. *Are there any that you or others don't let speak?*
A. The little ones; they're supposed to be quiet. They have Megan, she's eight, and she takes care of them. She has their vote, so she votes for them. They're not supposed to talk because they just cause trouble: they're noisy and they don't say anything that makes sense or is appropriate for what's going on. Mostly they're just asking for ice cream and things like that, so they're kind of useless at the meetings.

Q. *How long have you remembered these meetings taking place?*
A. I've only been invited to meetings for a couple of years.

Q. *Do you know that they took place before that?*
A. Yeah, because The Organizer keeps records.

Q. *Did she show you the records?*
A. Well, they talk about them all the time, 'cause they'll sit around and have arguments over who decided what and whose fault it was that we

did this thing instead of that thing. Then The Organizer will have to pull the records and tell everybody what happened. I knew about it because I knew she had the records from way back when. She was one of the people who came when we were eight, so I would guess that the meetings probably didn't start until we were about eight.

Q. *Did you know about the meetings then?*
A. I didn't know there were people then; I just heard voices.

Q. *Why do think that you started being invited to the meetings?*
A. Because my doctor said that I had to be.

Q. *When did you learn about the meetings?*
A. Probably about four years ago.

Q. *And why do think you started learning about the meetings?*
A. Because they'd tell me what they decided, what they voted that we were going to do in a particular situation. [Before that] we'd just do it and I wouldn't know why I had decided to do something.

Q. *Why do you think they started telling you?*
A. Because I was being a pain in the ass. I was complaining a lot that I didn't know what was going on and that I didn't know why I was doing things and why I wasn't doing things.

Samantha's inner democracy has probably been in place since her childhood and functions on any issue that might "cause problems" for Samantha's health, safety, financial security, and overall functioning. Now that Samantha, at her therapist's insistence, has been invited to participate, she too has a voice in her welfare and may discuss, argue, and vote. Her prior exclusion was not parts' malice, but the logical pre-therapy structure for a group of helpers whose original jobs entailed keeping a part in ignorance of events and whom Samantha knew only as voices. No One, whose sole job is to come out when all other parts of Samantha's mind are busy meeting inside, "is like a screen saver," Samantha says, subtly pointing out that even during important inner meetings, the body must continue to keep up appearances and cannot be allowed to look dissociated.

Samantha's inner organization resembles that of a small governing body with regular discussions, files of records, a voting process, and the equivalent of a "vice president" whose vote can break a tie. Here, Samantha gives an example of an organizational process during a personal crisis that endangered her children's health. In this internal process, the parts Cecelia and Julia play key roles.

> [My former husband] stopped paying his child support, and we didn't have any money. So Cecelia said, "Well hell, I know how to make money, I've done this before." I guess, to be honest, we all voted on it and let her do it because we didn't have any money and we had to feed the kids. So she picked up guys on the Internet and made money having sex with these guys. . . . [That went on] about three weeks. Then Dr. Russel said that if we didn't stop, he was going to commit us. [So] we had a meeting and everybody told Cecelia that we didn't want to go to the hospital and she had to stop. Julia said that she would go to the bishop at the church and tell him we didn't have any money and that he would help us. Cecelia wouldn't need to do that anymore. So that's what happened.

As Samantha knows, democracy does not guarantee a decision in the best interests of all. Partly because Cecelia thought nothing of getting money by continuing to do what has always been her job, the first vote brought an agreement that amounted to sacrificing the body's safety for the good of the children. Cecelia already knew how to make money because during her first marriage she had sold the body to pay for law school. Only after her therapist's threat of hospitalization did sweet, sensitive Julia think of using her role of "making people like us" to appeal to a bishop for help.

HOLDING BACK PARTS AND
THEIR MEMORIES

Since The Organizer's arrival, along with several other new parts, when Samantha was eight, The Organizer has been responsible for coordinating switches appropriate to the immediate demands of the outside world. Before that, as Samantha's The Smart One told me, switches were more haphazard: "It was just whoever wanted to be out was out, or whoever's job needed to be done was out." The addition of new parts seemed to necessitate an inner structure for the eight-year-old Samantha. In the outer world, the larger a working group, the more complex its organizational structure. So, it seems, may be the inner world: the larger a group of parts, the more efficient their organization if a woman is to be able to function. Having that organization fail can lead to consequences that range from confusing and embarrassing to job- or safety-threatening and a breakdown of functioning.

Child or adolescent parts whose main job is to hold abuse memories must be contained until they can be safely released. If they are let out in public, the change in behavior would be obvious. If they reveal their knowledge to the host before she is ready to work through each memory, their memories and their terror would disable the host or perhaps cause her suicide. Caroline, an accountant, told me that part of her mind writes in her journal, but when she is switched back to herself as the host, she is incapable of registering what is on the page. She tape-recorded her earliest therapy sessions because she could not remember them, but when she tried to listen to the tapes, her ears could hear but her mind was incapable of understanding what was said.

> Sometimes if I play the tape back, I can hear the words, but they stop at my ears; they don't register in my brain. Just like if one of us writes something that's not to be shared, I can see the words on the paper and I can read the words, but it's like it stops at my eyes, it doesn't go any

farther—unless we can make it go farther. It's very weird. But we were always like that.

Caroline's experiences are examples of the mind's ability to both know and not know about the past.

Elizabeth, a teacher, once heard an unsettling inner conversation that suggests that at least one part knows which traumatic memories have already been shared with Elizabeth as the host and which have not. Elizabeth reported, "I wasn't always informed. Does that make sense? I was very alarmed hearing conversations: 'No, don't tell her, she doesn't know that yet. No, she can't know that.' And me thinking, 'What don't I *know*?' being kind of pissed that I didn't know everything."

Elizabeth's other parts seem to be protecting her from knowing about experiences they think she as the host could not bear. Elizabeth still does not know or care to know some of her other parts and their experiences. She explains,

> After having memories, I thought there was the main part of me who knew [the] essence of things, but there were tons of things I didn't know. Now I accept that I don't need to know everything; I don't need to dig up and relive every single part. I have the sense of what happened and that's enough.

Elizabeth mentioned no inner meetings, but through the efforts of a part Elizabeth describes as her "cruise director," inner organization and appropriate switching are generally secured.

Elizabeth, Samantha, and Reba spoke of parts whose roles are to care for child parts. Elizabeth's The Good Mother tries to act as a mother to Elizabeth and to Elizabeth's child parts. The Good Mother seems to have a soothing rather than a disciplinary function for the young parts. Samantha and Reba, however, have parts whose specific jobs are to keep child and adolescent parts enclosed when their presence would be inappropriate or dangerous. Samantha's inner child-minder, Megan, helps ensure Samantha's daily functioning by restraining dangerous memories and behavior. When making important decisions, Megan makes sure that the youngest parts of Samantha's mind are also represented by a vote, keeping frustration and disorder at bay. Reba told me that one of her adult parts called Helper "kept all the other parts in their safe places inside until I was strong enough to be able to get [a therapist's] help." Like Elizabeth's unnamed part who warns other parts "she doesn't know that yet," Helper protected Reba from the release of traumatic memories until Reba, as the host, was ready to bear them and had found a therapist to help her do so. Helper has been with Reba since birth and "knows everyone inside and what happened to everyone," Reba says, making her an ideal minder and manager of traumatic memories. Currently, Helper continues to oversee the younger parts of Reba's mind during working hours so that her reputation and job security as a nurse are not endangered.

Where Parts Reside

We see rooms in our head, and that's where everybody goes. We can feel the changes in the body when they go in their room, 'cause it gets quiet.
—*Lucy, a forty-four-year-old social worker*

When parts hold meetings, vote, encounter each other and the host, hide, or are enclosed, where do these activities take place? Six of my interviewees—Ellie, Samantha, Caroline, Reba, Lucy, and Ruth—spoke of dwelling places for their parts where the parts stay when they are not controlling the body. Some of Ellie's other parts, for example, once resided in various parts of the body: the stomach, throat, hand, and the temple area of the head. Jesse, a part who lived in the throat, caused periodic pressure on the larynx, and Ellie would have breathing crises similar to asthma attacks. A part called Julie Ann resided in her stomach, periodically causing sharp stomach pains.

They were "hiding," Ellie said, but eventually made their presences known. Julie Ann, for example, first made herself known to Ellie, the host, by complaining loudly during Ellie's lunch break at work. Ellie, a retail manager, gave an amusing account of this first realization that some of her body pains might be caused by other parts of her mind:

> I had finished with my work, and at lunchtime I sat down to eat. And Julie Ann spoke to me for the first time. She said, "Hey, knock it off! I'm down here; quit throwing stuff on me." I said out loud, "Who said that?" And [a colleague] peeked around the corner of her office—'cause the lunchroom was right off of both of our offices—and she goes, "Who said *what*?" And I went, "Nothing, nothing." And that scared me that Julie Ann was actually talking out loud to me. I asked who it was—not out loud—I said, "Okay, who is this?" She said, "My name is Julie Ann," and I said, "Oh, and who are you?" And she said [in an impatient voice], "I'm *me*; I told you, I'm Julie Ann!" [Ellie and I laugh.] I said, "Where are you?" And she said, "I'm down *here*, quit throwing stuff on me." [She never used the word *stomach*,] I just got the sense that it was my stomach because I was eating at the time. I said, "I'm sorry; I didn't mean to throw things on you. You just move out of the way 'cause I'm hungry." So she did; and I finished eating and said, "Thank you."

The stomach was Julie Ann's choice of residence because that deep part of the body seemed to provide maximum safety and protection. Another part resided in the hands, especially the right hand, causing numbness. Ellie perceives a rationale behind this part's choice as well. The hands of abusers are instruments of love as well as of punishment, pain, and betrayal. Residing in the hands may have given that part of the mind a sense of control over the hands of others. Several parts resided in the temple area of the head, causing blinding headaches. Her therapist later helped Ellie use hypnosis to move all parts of her mind to the back of the brain, thus successfully eliminating the numbness in her hand, breathing crises, stomach pains, and headaches.

Ellie uses the terms "room" and "house" to describe where her parts now dwell, terms also used by Samantha, Reba, Lucy, and Ruth. All five women have dwelling places in their minds where their child parts can reside whenever they should not be seen or heard by the outside world. Ellie uses the term "children's room" as an analogy for an area of her mind. Ellie's obedient child parts allow themselves to be separated from other parts of Ellie's mind and confined to their "room" during times when a medical exam too much resembles past abuse. Only the mature parts of Ellie's mind who can distinguish between a gynecological exam and sexual abuse consciously enter the doctor's office.

> When I go to a gynecologist, it could be traumatic for some of the younger ones. I will say to them that they should stay in. And they're pretty good about that; they pretty much stay—it's really hard to explain—they stay within a certain area, I guess you'd call it. If you had to think of my brain as a little house, then they're staying in their own little room. And they don't open that door, it's locked. They don't come out until I leave [the doctor's office] and say, "You can come out now!" Then they can come out and be part of the rest of the group.

Similarly, Reba, a nurse, speaks of a "safe room" for her child parts, with her adult part Helper as child-minder to make sure that the noticeably different parts stay confined and quiet unless Reba is at home alone, with a trusted friend, or with her therapist. While the child parts are in the safe room, Reba cannot hear them. Several months after our interview, I wrote to Reba asking if she constructed her "safe room" on her own or with the help of a therapist. Reba wrote the following reply.

> As far as I know, we have always had "places" inside where the different child parts have hidden or gone to be safe. Helper was the one who decided that there needed to be one central area or place for the ones who started coming out of hiding to be gathered, where she could watch over and care for them. She tells me that she created the safe room

shortly before we started therapy. It started as one big room, but changed over time as we needed it to. Many "sleeping areas" were added on, as well as a meeting room, a playroom, and a playground, with swings, slide, etc. These areas are only accessible through the safe room so Helper has been able to control who can get in. Thus, the "children" can feel more secure that no one can get to them to harm them.

Reba's child parts do not realize that Reba's abusers can no longer harm her. Therefore, the origin of Reba's structure was the need for all parts of her mind to feel safe from abuse. Helper created "places" of safety for other parts so that Reba can function and pass as a singleton.

How "Rooms" Are Constructed

Lucy, a social worker, also has multiple dwellings where her "little ones" can feel safe, each in her or his own room. Lucy, as the host, constructed such dwellings on her therapist's advice because she previously had no structure inside and "it was a mess; everybody was everywhere . . . and it was noisy," as a part of Lucy's mind called Rose told me. Guiding the client in the creation of internal organization and structure is standard practice among skilled therapists who are well-versed in trauma and dissociation. Lucy's therapist talked to Lucy about how to organize her inner realm, then "we went in and everybody made their own space," Rose said. Lucy, with Rose and other parts, constructed in her mind a variety of "rooms" based on what each part envisioned as the safest from harm. Some rooms are under trees or in trees so that no one can reach them; some are soft and padded for extra protection. A few enterprising child parts constructed a playroom and a kitchen complete with a store of candy. When I asked Rose how she and other parts constructed their rooms, she described their process:

We had a meeting with everybody and said, "Okay, we've got to get the little ones to be safe," so we had to get some of the bigger ones to help us. We got them to help make what would feel good for them. So they got to design their own space using head pictures: we see rooms in our head, and that's where everybody goes. We can feel the changes in the body when they go in their room, 'cause it gets quiet. So, if somebody's really out of control, we say, "Okay, we need to have that one go to their room." At the beginning we'd have to sit down and really spend energy saying, "Okay, we're going to visualize this one going into its room and settling down." And then the body would settle down. Sounds pretty crazy, doesn't it? Explaining it's funny; I never explained it in this detail before.

Lucy's "head pictures" make the difference between the chaos of multiple homeless parts talking and screaming, and the orderly stillness made possible by visualized structures.

In Samantha's case, other parts seem to have created their rooms on their own, before therapy. The rooms were in place before Samantha, as the host, knew about them or had a room for herself inside her mind. Here she describes when, why, and how she constructed her own private dwelling place.

I think what happened was I had a stillborn baby and I didn't want to be here anymore. But my kids were all real upset, so I couldn't die. I wanted to just go away for a while. And I heard the voices telling me that I could: I just had to find somewhere to go, make a picture of it in my head, and it would be there. So I made a place that I could go to. [So,] now I have a room inside. [Or rather,] it's not really a room, it's more of a cabin. Then I went there and stayed for like a week. Before I came back, I kind of wandered around a little and saw some of the rooms they were in. [That was when I first became aware of the rooms] probably about five or six years ago.

Samantha designed a cabin in an idyllic setting, where she could take an inner vacation and escape from her sorrows and cares without dying. Her other parts told Samantha how easy it is to have such a soothing place. All she had to do was "make a picture of it" in her head, echoing Lucy's part Rose's description of using "head pictures" to "design" safe places within. Idyllic, soothing settings in nature, such as a beautiful meadow, appear to be popular retreats for the imagination as they are for reality. If the first identity becomes incapacitated by trauma early in life, she may remain in a meadow for years while other parts fully take over her functioning.[1] At times, the first identity may remain inside for a lifetime.[2]

Samantha's wise voices know what the mind can do and teach her how to "not be here," a protective capability reminiscent of Samantha's early ability to escape from her body, sit with her beloved doll, and watch her body on the bed during childhood abuse. After recently having laser surgery, and without physically leaving her bed, Samantha "went" to her lakeside cabin. I asked Samantha if she could feel herself there in the cabin, basing my question on my own paltry dissociative abilities. Samantha's reply, "I *was* there," revealed her surprise that I could have misinterpreted her words, and my incapacity to fully enter her world. When I asked Samantha where her dwelling places were, she replied simply, "In my head."

How Dwelling Places Look Inside

As Samantha mentioned, she, as the host, was not able to explore her complex inner structure until she first met the other parts of her mind and discovered their world. Samantha described her own, relatively new, dwelling place.

> [This place that I made for myself] is kind of like my room, but it's not a room, it's a place. Have you ever seen Lake Placid? It kind of looks like that except I've got a log cabin next to the lake, and it's really pretty and the air's all fresh and clean and cool—it's really nice. Sometimes when I want to, if none of the kids are home or if I can get away with it, I go there and I just relax.

Samantha's place is designed to be a retreat. Originally her place of recovery from the suicidal grief of having a stillborn child, Samantha now uses it during the rare times when she is free of her daily responsibilities and can relax. Her cabin contrasts with her description of the utilitarian structure for other parts of her mind, a structure that seems to combine elements of home and office.

> Everybody [has a room] except Megan because she stays in the room with the little ones: they all share a room. I can see [the others] in the hall or if I go to their room or the boardroom. I'll be doing something, and they'll call a meeting and I'll have to go. [They call a meeting in] lots of different ways. There's word-of-mouth: someone will just walk around and tell everybody that we're having a meeting—that's if it's not really important. Or, every room has a light panel, and one of the lights is a red light. If the red light goes on, that means there's an emergency meeting and you have to go to the boardroom right away. And since I'm not in my room very much, I hear like a beep, kind of a siren thing that goes off when my red light goes on so that I can know that there's a meeting and I'm supposed to go.

Many of the furnishings Samantha described are essential to her functioning. Because of a filing cabinet, for example, The Organizer can store Samantha's long-term memories and retrieve them as needed. The filing cabinet enables The Organizer to settle arguments among different parts about what happened in the past. When I asked Samantha to tell me or write about a typical incident of childhood abuse, it was The Organizer who wrote the account. The light panel assembles all parts so that Samantha can make important decisions with her whole mind.

Only one furnishing was installed at her therapist's suggestion. He recommended that Samantha include television sets for every room inside her mind. The television sets do not have programs for amusement or relaxation. They are closed-circuit sets for listening to and watching the body's speech and actions.

I can go to my room and leave the TV screen on. If I leave it on with the sound on, I can see and I can hear everything that's going on [outside]. We didn't always have TVs; the TVs started during therapy. My doctor told us that we should all, as much as we can, leave the TV screens on so that we know what's going on all the time.

With this one furnishing Samantha's therapist cleverly used his client's mental capabilities to "install" co-consciousness so that all of Samantha's mind is aware and informed even when not controlling the body.

The lawyer part of Samantha's mind, The Smart One, gave me an equally interesting account of Samantha's interior world. The Smart One has known that world from the inside far longer than Samantha has as the host. I had asked The Smart One if, during her law work, she knew when Samantha was paying attention. She replied that when she wanted to, she could go see Samantha and check on what she was doing. I asked how she did that, and she replied, "[I] just *go* there," with the implication "It's simple!" I explained that some description was necessary because not everyone knows how to do that, and she responded,

In what way I go there? Okay. Well, for Samantha, I go back inside, and she's got a special elevator that goes to her room. And so I go into her elevator, and I end up by myself 'cause not everybody is allowed to go to her room. And then it takes me to where her cabin is. And then I go find her [and] just check and see what she's doing, if she's got the TV on. Or I could just ask The Organizer whether she's got her TV on. [But I haven't always been able to check on Samantha.] Usually there was nothing to check on because she didn't have a place to go; she was just in abeyance when one of us was out. So, it's really only in the past few years that there's been anything to check on.

The Smart One's account adds more detail to Samantha's inner activity and structure. The Smart One, when free to go inside, has to take an elevator to reach Samantha's cabin, indicating that it is on a different level than the structure's other rooms. Furthermore, "not everybody is allowed" to enter Samantha's place in the mind, probably because their memories are considered too dangerous to come close to her. Also, her cabin was created as a later addition to the structure as a place of retreat. Her cabin's remoteness from the other parts' rooms and its exclusive status seem in keeping with the fact that Samantha, as the host, is the part of the mind previously entirely shielded from knowledge of traumatic events.

The Smart One's description of checking on Samantha also allows a peek into The Smart One's own room. "[When I'm not needed,] if I don't feel like paying attention, I can go back to sleep, read a book, watch a movie, or do whatever I feel like doing," The Smart One said. When she is not in control of the body and feels no need to pay attention to the outside world, The Smart One has her own leisure time to use as she pleases. She can simply "go back to sleep," suggesting the presence of a bed and of an ability to restore her energy when neither her advice from within nor her control are necessary. Evidently, her room is also stocked with a video player and books, which is logical because The Smart One presumably created and furnished the room herself with all that she, as the body's intelligence, requires for her edification and amusement.

Ruth, a physician, gave me a similarly thorough description of a highly structured interior world. Ruth calls it "a whole house inside my head." Her inner realm includes a tree house "for the kids" and a field. Other parts of Ruth's mind told her that the house has always been there, although as the host, Ruth does not have a room. "I don't really sleep—I mean, I sleep when the body sleeps, but [otherwise] I just sort of take care of everybody when I'm inside," she said. When not in control of the body, Ruth has a supervisory role, keeping other parts occupied so that they do not disturb a male part called The Physician, who is switched into control when Ruth enters her office. Ruth also often likes practicing medicine. "So if everybody's okay, then I hang out with The Physician and help with the sensitive side of things," she said. Ruth, who considers herself "not that good at decorating," described The Physician's bedroom as well as a meeting room in the "ten- or twelve-bedroom house."

The Physician has a centrally located room, and he always has his books. He also has an extra bed so that if one of the parts gets sick, [that part] will go in and sleep with The Physician because he is so strong that they feel he'll protect them. And he's got a really big desk where he sits and works late at night and goes over all the things he remembers about medicine. You know, a lot of times I read when I go to bed, and he's reading articles—well, it's hard to say: if I'm reading [medical articles] he's processing them. It's where I store my intelligence, my knowledge of medicine. I don't really like reading very much; The Physician likes to read, but he doesn't want to read anything but medical journals. [Ruth and I laugh.]

Then there is one big room with many chairs in a circle like a 12-Step meeting where everybody would get together and meet; a meeting of the minds, basically. That room is where the microphone for the head is if somebody wants to talk to me; and that's where the red button is for my ears ringing. They have a panic button they can push when they're upset. Like the other day it happened; I was coming back from work and my ears were ringing really loud. And I said, "What is it? What do you guys want?" They were remembering that I forgot to call my lawyer [and] they were trying to let me know.

Ruth's interior structure is uniquely hers, yet shares certain aspects with other women's interiors. Like Lucy, Ruth has built a tree house in which her child parts can play but also feel safe from the dangers they perceive as lurking on the ground. Ruth, Samantha, and Reba have a meeting room in which votes are taken and decisions made, and outdoor areas for relaxation or play. The greatest similarities are those between Ruth and Samantha, who have three more items in common. Both women have signal systems of light and/or sound: while Samantha hears a "beep" or "siren" signal, Ruth hears ringing in her ears. For both women, the color red signifies immediate emergency communication. Both of them have a multileveled structure for dwellings, although Ruth has yet to explore the first floor to see what she might find.

Like Samantha and Elizabeth, Ruth has a part who coordinates switching. However, Ruth alone spoke of a "switching room" where Ruth or other parts go to alternately take control of the body. Here, Ruth describes herself, as the host, being switched into control:

> There's this switching room where—it's a big machine like in "Star Trek." It had a control room. [A] part called The Caretaker would push the button for the switching and you walk into sort of like a tube: it's a tall, glassed-in kind of area. And it [has] a door that looks like a person, and you walk through it. And then you go from being really tiny in your head to feeling the body. I remember I would feel—it's like if you were to take a balloon and blow it up to the right height and width.

"Tiny" in her head when not in control, Ruth seems to describe swelling in height and width until she can comfortably fill and feel her whole body. The room that effects this transformation appears to be based on Star Trek technology but is also reminiscent of Alice in Wonderland's bottled potions for quickly changing her size.

Ruth's "switching room" is her imaginative construction of psychobiological events related to switching. The room illustrates the observation that the center of the body's control appears to have a "location" in the body/mind. Accordingly, when a person has dissociated parts of the mind, only the part in the specific location for control would be able to take charge of the body.[3] Ruth uses fantasy representations familiar from television and books to picture this center of control and organize the events unfolding in her mind.

A "Room" Underground. In contrast to Ellie, Samantha, Reba, Lucy, and Ruth, Caroline did not specifically mention rooms, though she spoke of parts' meetings and safe places inside, suggesting that she sees interior structures. She did, however, describe an interesting underground structure for deeply buried parts of her mind. One such buried part is Macey, who came when Caroline's father put her at the mercy of a group of men who "played

dress-up." Macey took this abuse and kept the memories. Caroline recounts
a part called Vicki bringing the buried part Macey to the surface:

> For Macey there was a period of time with a whole set of male people.
> It was like going to this man's house, and there were two other men there
> that things happened with. It was all like playing dress-up and stuff like
> that. But [my father] was around; he was probably in the other room.
> That's really bad, [but] we know about it now because Vicki brought
> Macey out of the tunnel. When we were going through therapy and
> needing to deal with everyone, Vicki said there were people in the tun-
> nel that needed to come out. And so she went into the tunnel and
> brought Macey out. Nobody really wanted her to, but she did it any-
> way. [Macey] couldn't communicate, so she just stayed with me and
> with [another part called] Pam, [and] depressed the shit out of us. She
> didn't really talk, she just lay there, and so it was very depressing to be
> around her. [In therapy] we planned the time when we would wake her
> up in a really safe setting. We led up to that day, and then we had a dou-
> ble session; a whole afternoon. And after that was over, [my therapist]
> didn't have anybody else for the day. His office was in his home, and we
> just stayed in his office. He went upstairs and did other stuff and would
> just come check on us every once in a while.

Caroline describes the part Vicki disclosing to Caroline, as the host, and
her therapist a heretofore secret place underground where some parts reside
who "need to come out" in the context of therapy. Vicki then brings out
the evidently prostrate Macey against the will of the other parts who do not
want Macey around them. Bringing Macey's memories to their level
depresses Caroline and some of her other parts before they know why. This
is a visual depiction of a traumatic memory that reveals itself as unexplained
feelings, pictures, or body sensations before it can be put into words. Wisely,
Macey is not willing to speak until Caroline's therapist makes special
arrangements for supervising her safety. Caroline's is an account of a part
who holds memories so abhorrent that the part must be contained in a "tun-

nel," a level separate from and deeper than some other parts and their memories. Caroline's graphic interior structure gives a traumatic memory a place in her mind where it can lie hidden for over forty years until the time is right for coming to the surface and being put into words.

THE IMPORTANCE OF HAVING INNER ORGANIZATION

My interviewees' accounts reinforce the importance of inner organization to help a mind in dissociated parts function as smoothly as possible, avoid suicide, and pass as "normal." Some organizational form, from the simple and basic to the extensive and elaborate, was common among my interviewees. Gabbi alone mentioned no such form at the time of the interview, nor had she any communication with other parts of her mind. She was struggling the most of all my interviewees from other parts taking control of the body at inappropriate times.

My interviewees illustrate some of the mind's possible organizational techniques. To organize various parts, the mind naturally uses the familiar, just as it does to visualize identities. Parts gather to discuss and make decisions, imitating teams of people in the outside world who must live or work in concord. Familiar, tangible architecture provides the images for inner habitats. As long as information must be blocked, "walls" and "ceilings" help separate other parts from the host and perhaps from each other. "Safe rooms" confine traumatic memories during stressful events, while "meeting rooms" enable separated parts to work together and reach decisions. "Switching rooms" help the mind shift smoothly from one part to another, and cabins in idyllic settings offer escape from life's stresses. These structures serve to organize numerous parts of one person's mind just as tangible architecture helps organize numerous people.

Internal architecture is tailor-made for the mind's needs. Therefore the number of parts, their ages, and their roles are likely to determine the number, placement, and extent of parts' dwellings. Parts' ages and characteristics also determine a room's contents: books for the intellectual part, a filing cabinet for the part who stores and files memories, swings and candy for child parts. Because inner structures are created according to need, they can evolve architecturally as those needs change. Bedrooms are added, as are conference rooms, playrooms, cabins, playgrounds, and beautiful scenery.

The needs of the youngest parts are particularly vital. They are emotionally and cognitively children in constant fear of their abusers. Their need to feel protected is paramount. At the same time, mature parts must be sure that child parts refrain from controlling the body in public, especially at work. Inner walls confine the child parts and help them feel safe. Therefore, some of the "safe places" inside a woman's mind serve the dual purpose of protecting both the youthful and the mature parts of the mind.

My interviewees illustrate that inner structures do not automatically exist for parts, nor do all people who have parts create such structures. However, a traumatized child's early experiences of being outside the body and watching it possibly encourage the establishment of "places" within the mind. Barbara told me that during childhood abuse, she would start to feel mainly the physical pain and some emotions, then would be taken out of her body by angels to a "nice place" from where she would see "the other girl" on the bed. Barbara describes herself as "not a visual person," but since those early years she has had what she calls a "nowhere place," which she does not visualize, but which she nonetheless considers a place to which she, as the host, sometimes goes.

The impetus to create a more structured interior comes from some parts themselves or from a trusted person outside. The imagination then creates structures according to the mind's requirements either on its own or with a therapist's guidance. In order to establish such structures, one or more mature parts can assist those parts that remain in the helplessness of childhood. Lucy and Reba illustrated that their mature parts either created the inner architecture alone or helped child parts create the internal spaces they need.

Such inner structures can range from the simple and utilitarian, to as comfortable and elaborate as imagination can make them. Architecture and furnishings can help the mind be prepared for any contingency. Everything from elevators to personal beepers can grace these interiors, whose purpose is to offer security, safety, privacy, or companionship and provide whatever spaces, furniture, and technology parts deem necessary to avoid chaos and encourage order, concord, and efficiency.

Parts other than the host may be the best sources of information about their dwelling places. They sometimes create their structures without the host, who learns of them years after the fact. Samantha, as the host, learned about her interior structure only when she desperately required one for herself as a place for "going away" without dying. Only on returning from her own place did she wander around inside her mind and see the rooms her other parts had been constructing since at least her eighth year. Ruth, as the host, was told by other parts that the house inside her head has "always been there. I drew it in '96 or '97 and became aware of it then," she said, illustrating how the act of drawing a picture can be a way other parts share information with the host. During her description of her inner house, other parts of Ruth's mind were evidently listening and occasionally correcting Ruth, as when Ruth said, "Jack and The Aristocrat share a room . . . oh no, they said they don't. Okay, Jack has his own room." The part of Lucy called Rose described the creation of the places inside her mind. Rose was the part of Lucy's mind who spoke whenever the interview turned to events inside the mind. Lucy explained that Rose and other parts are more knowledgeable about their interior world than is Lucy who, as the host, is out and controlling the body much of the time.

Although parts' organization is an essential asset, it does not necessarily protect a woman from periodic loss of functioning or suicide attempts, though it may reduce the incidence of such crises. Other parts of Samantha's mind helped Samantha "go away" without dying, and a published account tells of inner "community meetings" for all parts to agree not to attempt suicide.[4] A therapist can use the client's skill in creating "head pictures" as part of therapy. For example, Lucy organized her mind after learning about such possible organization from her therapist. Samantha's therapist skillfully instructed Samantha to include closed-circuit television as part of her inner furnishings so that all parts of Samantha's mind can see and hear what the body is doing even when they are not in control. When I last spoke with Barbara, years after the original interview, she had just begun creating some inner architecture with the help of her therapist. She especially wants an enclosure for her child parts during working hours. Barbara has always had the sensation of having compartments in her head and considers these compartments the feeling of having a mind in parts. She considers visualized rooms in a house as logical extensions of a compartmentalized mind.

Possibly the type of abuse, the number of parts, the choice of profession, or innate imaginative tendencies singly or together influence a person's inner organization. It is interesting that Samantha, a lawyer, and Ruth, a physician, described exceptionally elaborate organizational techniques and structures, even though some professional women's parts have efficient inner organization without inner architectural structures. Despite these variations, my interviewees suggest that, to varying degrees, people with minds in parts are artists, visualizing people, places, and objects with the skill and vividness of painters or novelists. The artistry of a mind in parts, however, is born of traumatic experiences and invisible to the outside world.

Points to Keep in Mind

- A major reason for internal structure is the need to keep child parts enclosed when necessary and to give them a sense of safety from harm.

- If parts do not have a system of internal organization and structure, such a system is a goal to consider discussing with a therapist.

- Although some people function well without inner architecture for their parts, such architecture seems to greatly help those who have it.

5

THE WORKDAY
WITH PARTS

I like to get to work before other people to get a sense of what happened the day before . . . and see if anything's missing during that time that I may have to deal with. I do spend a lot of time trying to think if I can remember the whole day before.

—*Gabbi, a forty-two-year-old director*
in the field of medical research

Once in a while, one of my others will come out while I'm at work. I just excuse myself from what I'm doing if it's an okay moment, and I go in the bathroom and just sit there and remind them, "Hey, this is my work. You can't be out."

—*Reba, a thirty-two-year-old nurse*

I can remember going to the office and sitting down; I just can't remember the law work I did there. [But] I know that things were getting done.

—*Samantha, a forty-three-year-old lawyer*

◉

Imagine a workday in which you often cannot remember what you did the day before; or you have to take all your children with you to the workplace; or you have no idea how to do your own job. These are experiences for Gabbi, Reba, and Samantha, respectively, every working day. Each of their lives illustrates a different type of work experience. Gabbi and Reba are both the host identities and are also in charge of work outside the home. However, Gabbi is in the early stages of getting to know her other parts and of gaining their cooperation, keeping her in constant uncertainty about what has and will happen at work. Reba's other parts, in contrast, are in close communication with Reba and with each other and generally obey Reba so that she and they are more like a team, all parts of one mind working together. Unlike Gabbi and Reba, Samantha is a cohost but not the worker. Another part of her mind pursues the profession of law. Each woman has her unique story to tell, and these stories, combined with the experiences of other women, form a complex view of the effects of dissociated identities on women's professional lives.

GABBI: COPING WITH UNCERTAINTY AND FORGETFULNESS

In my experience [having parts] has been an impediment and difficulty in the workplace. When you're constantly living with the question, "What did I do yesterday? What am I going to do today?" it becomes much more critical when you're in the workplace. People don't expect you to have an off day or a weird day or do something very odd. Because I'm a director and a manager, [I'm] in a visible position, constantly watched and looked at and having that hanging over my head all the time.

Gabbi is a director in the field of medical research in charge of finance, human resources, administration, and building maintenance. Her role is motivating, training, and mentoring her staff, whom she manages and coordinates, making sure they have what they need and that all the work is done.

The tense helplessness her other parts cause at the workplace became apparent as soon as Gabbi began to speak about her workdays. Gabbi described the working life of a competent, well-trained professional, confident in her capabilities as finance and human resource manager in medical research but battling for control of her consciousness.

> I'm always worried about when I have meetings scheduled, if I'm going to be okay. Is it going to be a good day, a bad day, an easy day, or a not easy day? How much energy am I going to be using just maintaining control, and how much do I have to do for my job? In my previous job I did a lot of presentations to boards of directors. Public speaking was never anything I wanted to be doing, so that was a stressful thing anyway. And then to always have the knowledge that no matter how much I could prepare or control everything and do the best I can, I know there's things that I can't control and there's times I could switch [and] I have no ability to affect that. So I constantly felt like if I switched at the wrong time and to a child it would be a problem. And most of mine are very young, clearly inappropriate in the workplace, literally not able to function, and certainly not able to function at the level of my position. I always knew it could mean I wouldn't have a job the next day.

Gabbi's other parts remain aloof from her and largely uncommunicative. She perceives them as being solely a disadvantage at work and bringing no advantages. Indeed, having a traumatic past and a mind divided into parts changed the course of her career: she would have liked to have become a doctor but feared that the stress of medical school would be so great as to threaten her ability to function.

During the interview, Gabbi described a typical working day as beginning with anxiety and ending prematurely by "losing" the afternoon because another part had taken control. Her worries and fears include a constant uncertainty about what has or might happen at work, and her visibility at work increases her unease. The fear of being switched to another part is with her at every business meeting or public speaking engagement knowing, as she does, that such a switch could mean losing her job and her financial security.

Some of Gabbi's other parts do take over at the workplace, and Gabbi is occasionally switched without coworkers noticing anything unusual. When Gabbi goes around asking staff how they are, this simple morale-boosting is a responsibility an adolescent part sometimes carries out quite well.

> You can go have lunch with people in any kind of state of being, and it's not very obvious. Most people want to talk about their situation and themselves, so as long as you're there listening, they're not really in tune to you. They have no idea where you are and what your state of mind is. They're talking about themselves, so you sit there and listen. And even if I have no idea what they've said, I think their perception is that I'm always there and that I really care about them.

However, at times, peers have recognized significant changes or become confused about inconsistencies in the way Gabbi behaves. "Sometimes [my voice changes but] largely, from what people tell me, I think it's more subtle than that: it's more a change of vocabulary, a change in demeanor." She has been switched at meetings, and this was part of the reason why she left her last job where she had worked almost sixteen years. "I was going through a difficult time—I was hospitalized twice—and it became more and more difficult to maintain control." After one such meeting, one of the directors asked her what the matter was, saying that Gabbi had spoken inappropriately or had not talked about the topic on the agenda. The director was concerned that Gabbi was addicted, thinking that what she saw as "radical mood changes" were drug-induced.

> I also got reprimanded a couple of times from my boss [during] the last couple of years [at that job]: verbal warnings, written warnings about things that I said I was going to do [and] didn't do. I didn't show up to one board presentation: that's a major screw-up. [Also,] I remember we had a lunch meeting about some budget things. I was unprepared and I guess, at one point, said something that my boss, who was the presi-

dent of the organization, took as an insult to him—and so that's it for getting in trouble. He said he was quite surprised, that he thought he had known me in the eight years we had worked together and never expected anything like that. I apologized. I said I had no explanation for what I did. I toyed a while with telling him. He knew that there was something going on in my life 'cause I had been hospitalized. [But] I never told him what that was; he was never anybody I was comfortable could handle the information.

Gabbi was faced with an insolvable problem: how can a woman with a mind in parts explain embarrassing, insulting, uncharacteristic behavior to a director without disclosing the truth? Because of the stress, pressure, and politics of her eighty-hour week at that job, and the cumulative problems related to having parts, Gabbi eventually left, turned down equivalent jobs, and took a pay cut and fewer responsibilities in order to have time and energy for self-care and therapy.

Gabbi is now director of finance and administration for a management group that conducts clinical trials. She has only thirty staff as opposed to the seventy-five of her former job, and a smaller budget to manage, but a different type of stress has come with this job: high turnover and an unhappy and complaining staff looking for jobs. Gabbi describes how the feelings of being overwhelmed and having no control over events thrust a woman back into childhood:

> I start getting more emotional 'cause I want them to be happy and there's not a whole lot I can do about it, [and] I start feeling out of control, that there's nothing I can do. It's reminiscent of my past. The more it hits on anything that's emotional, that is any way related to my own past, the more vulnerable I get.

This is a common theme among my interviewees: workplace stress recalls abusive situations. Naturally, when such feelings begin, other parts of Gabbi's mind perceive that it is time to take control of consciousness.

Responding to perceived threat is and always was their job. Vulnerability also has to do with balancing energy: the more energy Gabbi, as the host, must give other people, and the more energy she needs for herself, the less she can control the switching. She voices the recurring theme that energy is needed to monitor emotions and to try to keep other parts of the mind inside, and this needed energy is often consumed by long working hours, the work itself, and workplace-related emotions. When Gabbi is switched at work, she can lose anywhere from an afternoon to weeks of time. "[Then] I'm back and don't know what's gone on." At the time of the interview, the longest recent switch was about a week and a half. Because of the continued switching, Gabbi begins the day by seeing if she can remember the day before or if blocks of time are missing that she may have to reconstruct. If she can remember most of the day before and feels comfortable inside, she can go ahead and work. But at times, Gabbi is on edge, her mind is not clear, and every ounce of her strength is used to stay present and focused.

> I have dialogues with myself now, saying, "You're okay, it's the year 2000, you're at work, you've got ten minutes to do this," to try to keep myself in a schedule or routine. When I'm functioning like that, I'm really vulnerable to switch: the more energy I'm expending that way, the less energy I have to hold off other parts taking over. So as I get weaker, they get stronger.

Sometimes Gabbi's other parts do not go to work at all when in control, causing Gabbi's partner to notify the therapist, who tries to bring Gabbi back into control to protect her job. When her other parts do go to work, not much work is done. Gabbi is unclear about which part of her mind goes to work when she does not. She thinks that a part called Heather may have some limited abilities at work, but that the other parts are unable to do anything other than have general conversations. Fortunately, Gabbi's current boss is not demanding and gives Gabbi much latitude about her work; and because Gabbi hires competent staff, they largely take care of themselves and can go a week or two without Gabbi's help. Some of Gabbi's work entails sitting in her office at her computer, an activity easy to mistake as work when actually nothing useful is being done.

"I Knew It Would Not Have Been Accepted"

In spite of her other parts' frequent appearances at work, Gabbi has never lost a job because of them. Her staff and employer do not recognize them as separate identities and do not realize that at times, the forty-two-year-old director they perceive as working at her computer is controlled by a teenage part of her mind playing computer games. Rough edges do appear, however. If she is switched before completing a piece of work, another part hands in work that is wrong or incomplete, and Gabbi has been called in later to explain herself and redo the work. Staff members have noticed marked differences in her behavior, and one made the telling remark, "You didn't seem yourself yesterday." Fear of such incidents causes Gabbi to isolate herself from collegial contact, an isolation she feels and regrets.

> I'm probably less involved with people at this job than I was at the previous job; more deliberate in staying at arm's length. I'm less open, less available, [and] I don't socialize. Nobody really knows about my life.

At a recent evaluation, Gabbi knew that her boss did not understand why Gabbi reacted or said things that were so unexpected. She felt the need to explain herself to him. Yet, bettering her relationship with her boss or staff through explanation and disclosure seems out of the question.

> I don't think it's a safe place to go; I don't think that many people can understand it. If I was forced to, I don't know what I would do. I left my last job rather than address the situation. I could have stayed at my other job, but I had a period where I would have been disabled. So I would have had to explain a whole lot more, and I knew it would have

changed everything; . . . I knew it would not have been accepted, understood, [or] kept confidential. And I didn't want to be there for that change.

If she ever did disclose, Gabbi would want listeners to understand and respect the information without having it cloud their opinion of her or behavior toward her. In reality, the opposite has occurred.

I have no doubt that if my direct bosses in either my previous job or now knew, that it would have a serious effect on—everything: what they invested me with; what work they felt comfortable giving me; just uncertainty about [my] capabilities. . . . I'm not sure anything can overcome that [stigma]. I had been fifteen years in my previous job, had a glowing work record; I was audited by outside firms and Medicare constantly, [and] those reviews were always very good. But after fifteen years, when I had some very rough couple of months and was hospitalized, my job [and] my abilities came into question. It was like none of what I had done mattered . . .[and my boss] felt like he couldn't trust anything from there forward—not even knowing the whole story! He [just] knew it was a psychiatric hospitalization, and that was enough for him. It didn't matter that there had been fifteen years before that; he felt I couldn't be trusted, I couldn't be counted on, that he couldn't continue to give me responsibility because if he did, it would be too much pressure and send me over the edge.

Gabbi's Possible Future

Gabbi is working hard to minimize her other parts' negative impact at work. One of her biggest fears is that at some point they will become unmanageable and interfere with her employment to the point of disability. "I support myself . . . [and it's] always in the back of my mind that I could become unable to work."

Although her day-to-day struggle leaves Gabbi little peace to think about future work or changes in career, she is considering returning to school to get a doctorate in psychology and becoming a counselor. She has to weigh many possibilities: Will a new job cause more stress and therefore impede the healing process? Would her experiences with psychological distress be more a help or a hindrance as a practicing counselor? "I go back and forth: on good days I think I have a lot to offer having been through a lot of it. And on tough days I feel like I [can] barely take care of myself, so how could I possibly help anybody else." Nonetheless, Gabbi is undaunted enough to consider a career change and, indeed, the professional success of Barbara and Lucy, the two counselors who have parts, should be encouraging. Gabbi's achievements in therapy are likely to gradually help her at work whether or not she decides to change her career. Whatever her decision, she can pride herself on her overall excellent work record and managerial, self-supporting status in spite of formidable obstacles.

REBA: KEEPING HER TEAM TOGETHER

During the first couple of years after I graduated from college and I—we—were getting into therapy with a good therapist, it was really hard maintaining a job, especially in the early stages of therapy. There were times when I would remember getting up to get ready for work, but then I wouldn't remember *going* to work. And then I would find out that one or the other had called in to my work and told them that I was sick and wasn't going to be coming in. I was worried about being able to keep a job and [having] other people find out that I had these other parts in me because I was scared that they would think I was crazy and not want to be around me. And also not knowing what was going on during different periods of time, like there could be days at a time that I wouldn't know what had happened or where I'd been, or who I'd talked to, or anything. I just felt like I had no control.

Reba is a registered nurse who graduated from college with a bachelor of science degree in nursing. Like Gabbi, Reba is the part of her mind who is the worker, and at the time of the interview was employed as a registered nurse in an office with six obstetrician/gynecologists. She takes medical histories from patients; prepares patients for exams; assists with exams; schedules surgeries; obtains and handles lab specimens; and does telephone triage with patients who call in with questions and concerns.

As she describes them, Reba's earliest working experiences sound very much like Gabbi's, as do her experiences with work-related stress. Reba's first job was in a cardiac care unit to which patients came directly from intensive care. "There was so much stress going on with work and with therapy that it was hard to keep even the motivation to *go* to work. I would go home crying; I would get up crying; I felt like I was stuck in a situation I was never going to get out of." Reba felt trapped, and newly retrieved memories and feelings brought the wish to die. She attributes her continued functioning at work during that volatile time to her therapist's determination. Reba finally did have to leave her job at the hospital because, like Gabbi, she found the combination of intense therapy and highly stressful work too explosive to bear.

Her next job as a home health nurse was easier on her. Although the responsibility of being a case manager for a large group of patients was great, she enjoyed the self-sufficiency: "[I]t was just me and my patient." Most of her patients were elderly and diabetic, and Reba taught them how to take care of themselves in their homes so that they would not have to go to a nursing home. The sometimes long drive from one patient to another meant that Reba spent considerable time in her car, and during that time she thought about the work being done in therapy with her other parts. "And sometimes, as long as they let me drive safely and didn't try to take over, I would let them talk to me while I was driving. And that helped." Reba's words reveal that by then she, as the host, had gained insight into and control over her other parts. Realizing their need to speak and be listened to and "letting" them talk to her shows that she was capable of setting limits on the extent of their presence during working hours. She continued intense work in therapy, where memories and feelings were told, believed, and discussed. Helpful inner changes took place such as all parts' increased cooperation on mutual goals and their understanding of the need for Reba's work. Reba's two other adult parts help Reba keep her child parts from disrupting work, an important factor in the smooth professional functioning of women with child parts.

Since Reba has begun working with obstetrician/gynecologists, she has been well-treated and appreciated, and workplace problems with her other parts have lessened. When she gets ready for work in the morning, sometimes there is switching, but Reba is now more aware of her internal life and able to keep enough control to leave home on time. As a working woman, Reba now feels the advantages of six years of therapy specifically addressing dissociated identities and of having two adult parts of her mind called Circle and Helper who are active, mature assistants. Obstetrics and gynecology are, however, the medical specialties that most resemble childhood sexual abuse, and therefore pose a special challenge to any woman with a past like Reba's, part of which she recounted in Chapter 3. Consequently, Reba has established an inner space like a child's room for her child parts, a space that Reba calls "the safe room." But just as children now and then burst out of their rooms even when a child-minder is present, so Reba's inner safe room is not entirely foolproof.

> Usually, when I'm at work, Helper has them in the safe room. [But] there have been a few times when some of the ones inside wouldn't come all the way out but they'd look out; they'd watch to see what was happening, and they'd have their questions about what was going on. Or, sometimes when I had to go in the room with the doctor when he was doing a pelvic exam on a woman, they'd get upset. And as soon as I was able to, I'd have to go to the bathroom and close the door and quietly talk with them and let them know, "This is okay; the doctor is not hurting the woman, the doctor is taking care of her and making sure she's healthy and the baby's healthy." Just helping them to know that what the doctors were doing in the exams was not the same thing as what

happened to us with the abuse. I get them back in the safe room and [then] we talk about it more after we get home.

Reba's silent reassurances are examples of her repeated attempts to bring other parts out of their state of self-defense and into the realm of a safe, normal life.

When Reba has to assist with minor surgery such as dilation and curettage, the sight of the blood and instruments triggers abuse memories for Reba and for some of her other parts, requiring a simultaneous effort for Reba as a nurse and as a "mother" of child parts. While she assists in the surgery, she silently tries to reassure and contain the parts frozen in childhood: "Please go back in the safe room, let me handle this. We'll talk about it in a little while." Then she calls for one of her inner child-minders to make sure that child parts are in the safe room until she completes the surgery and assists the patient in recovery. When she is the late-shift nurse, she alone has to stay behind after surgeries to clean the instruments and the room, getting everything ready for the next day. As soon as the doctor leaves, Reba goes into one of the already clean rooms and talks with the upset parts to try to calm them so that she can finish the cleaning and preparation. At one point, such surgical assistance caused an inner rebellion against continuing work and Reba had to see her therapist that very night. Reba pleaded with other parts, "This is the best job I've had; I don't have to work evenings, weekends, holidays; I don't have to be on call all the time; . . . and I like it. It's a good environment, and good benefits." She also presented them with a subtle threat: if they wanted to remain safe from her parents and have therapy, she had to work, because otherwise she would not be able to afford rent and food and would have to return to her parents' house.

Since that crisis, Reba says, her younger parts have been more cooperative about not coming out or even "peeking out" when she is working so that she can remain focused entirely on her work. Once in a while however, parts will still try to come out at work, but Reba thinks that she catches any switching at work before changed speech or behaviors give her away. Nowadays, she is more aware of other parts' attempts to come out because she can sense their coming, like sensing that someone is approaching from behind. At the next opportune moment, she excuses herself, goes into the bathroom, and reminds them, "Hey, this is my work. You can't be out. You need to go back in the safe room." She then promises to take care of them when she gets home. "I don't get angry or yell at them, I just talk with them." Like a good mother, she is patient and understanding with the younger parts of her mind, explaining her work to them and making sure that they are rewarded for quiescence at work with time to control the body and pursue their own interests after working hours.

"I Don't Tell Them"

Reba does not mind having child parts at work as long as they stay in the safe room. She does, however, get flustered and frustrated when they come out while she is working because she fears disclosing the truth about any changes in voice or behavior. "I don't want people that I work with to know, partly because I worry that I will lose my job, that they won't understand, that they won't trust me anymore around the patients." As a result, Reba, like Gabbi, is reticent with her colleagues and intentionally vague with her answers to personal questions:

> I'm afraid to reveal too much about myself, you know? It might get into a conversation where I would have to explain myself more. I've always felt like I have to hide who I really am from other people; I have to hide us, I have to hide the fact that I have multiple personalities, because they won't understand [and I don't want them] to suddenly be afraid of me or not want me around them.

Reba has, however, defended others. When fellow nurses criticized a formerly abused patient terrified of a gynecological exam for "carrying on" in the doctor's office, Reba tried to explain the patient's behavior. She also notified authorities when she learned that her parents were trying to take in a foster child, even though she knew that her parents might try to avenge themselves by calling her supervisor and causing Reba to lose her job. She revealed her childhood abuse and explained the situation to her supervisor who said, "I've seen your work, I've seen how good you are. I trust you and I know that if somebody calls and says horrible bad things about you, that they're not going to be telling me the truth." This response was warmly appreciated by all parts of Reba's mind.

Nonetheless, Reba shies away from the idea of disclosing her separate identities to her supervisor. "I don't think that she would understand. I would *hope* that she would still be okay with me, because I've worked there a little over a year now [and] she has seen how I work. . . . But I don't know; I just worry that people won't understand and they'll think that I'm crazy or they'll be scared of me, so I don't tell them." Reba is also not certain that her supervisor would keep a disclosure to herself and is especially afraid that the doctors in the office would no longer trust her to take care of their patients if they knew the truth. "Even though I've worked there for this length of time and they've told me that I'm a good nurse, that I'm good in the office, I still worry that it would change their opinion of me." Ideally, Reba would want a disclosure to change nothing about her excellent work record or her relationship with office staff members. "[I'd want them to] still accept me as I am, and know that it's not going to be detrimental to my job performance and that I'm not going to do or say anything that's going to harm anybody." She realizes, however, that this ideal is unlikely and that, like Gabbi, she could have many more years of a flawless work record erased by a single disclosure.

SAMANTHA: SOMEONE ELSE DOES THE JOB

[In my law office while the law work was being done] I was looking at this really pretty tree out my window, and I was thinking how neat this was and how cool it was. And I was going into [my second husband's] office and giving him hugs—and daydreaming.

Samantha, as the sum of her parts, is a lawyer specializing in bankruptcy law. In contrast to both Reba and Gabbi, however, Samantha, as a cohost, is not the part of her mind who is the worker, as she explained in Chapter 1. She is conscious during working hours, however, and can watch or look out the window while The Smart One, the name of the part who performs all intellectual activities, is busy being a lawyer, assisted by a part called Julia whose job is to be nice to clients. Samantha is an example of people who have two or more parts who divide the requirements of a job among themselves and may see themselves as a group or family.[1] When I was interviewing Samantha by telephone and began to ask about work outside the home, The Smart One was switched into control, unbeknownst to me. I was aware of the switch only when The Smart One introduced herself. "This is The Smart One. [I was switched out] because you were asking about things that had to do with legal work." The Smart One sounds like Samantha except for a confident, abrupt manner of speaking, as opposed to Samantha's tentative gentleness. This is not surprising since The Smart One is the purely intellectual part of Samantha's mind. Despite the identical voice, The Smart One has a will of her own, as illustrated by this verbatim excerpt of my interview with her in which she mainly speaks of herself in the first person plural and repeatedly refers to discussions or arguments with other parts.

The Smart One's Perspective

"Samantha's father wanted us to get a degree in library science, so we got a master's degree in library science and worked at a science library. I did that [with] Julia.

"Then we did nothing for about two years while we raised kids. [I] started law school after Ben was born because I'd had it: Samantha and Julia were folding laundry and watching soap operas, and there was no way that I was going to sit around while they were watching soap operas. I just went and got an application and applied [to law school].

"We started going to law school at night so we could still take care of the children during the day. And that worked pretty well until our ex-husband got mad. He was in charge at night, but they were pretty calm at night. But there were about twenty minutes when he got home from work where things were hectic, and he couldn't stand it. So he told us we had to switch to day classes so that we could watch the kids at night when he was home. So we switched to day classes and worked out schedules that would minimize the amount of time the children were with babysitters and did all our studying at night after the children had gone to sleep so that it didn't take away time from the children or from him.

"And we wound up doing really well in law school—I did really well—and got a super job. But it was very time-consuming: jobs with major firms take a lot of time. So that made it difficult, but I kept the job for about eight years, and then got another one. Eventually, I had to quit working for large law firms and had to be on my own because it was too complicated trying to get everything done while I had an office that I had to be at, set times that I was supposed to be there. [That's when I decided to work from home.]

"I do all the legal work and [Julia does] the hand-holding and being nice to people. [I always know what Julia is doing and vice versa.] Julia and I both have a lot of stamina, so when you put us together we're a pretty good team. When you have some of the others out at the same time watching, or trying to participate, or making comments, or somehow involving themselves in what's going on, then we get tired more easily and it's harder to accomplish what we wanted to do.

"[I think that work] is easier [when you have parts] because different people do their own job and you always have the right person doing the right job. You don't have somebody doing it who doesn't know what they're doing. [But] sometimes it's difficult because you can't concentrate as you would like to because of people [inside] talking in the background or people getting scared by aggressive attorneys. For example, if there was a very aggressive attorney on the other side who was yelling and screaming at us, they would panic [and] it would be hard for me to stay in control.

"I think when I'm taking a lot of clients it makes [the others inside] feel left out or unimportant because their role is minimized and my role is much more important. So I think that's hard on them. There really aren't ways to get around it because I can't involve them in my work any more than they are; I can't have them doing things that they're not able to do. And when I'm working for a client, I have to be focused on what the client's needs are and I can't be fussing with them and trying to make them feel better about whether they're important or not when I've got work to do."

As The Smart One tells us, before she became a lawyer, the need to please Samantha's father was the driving force behind career decisions, then work outside the home ceased when motherhood intervened. The Smart One put her foot down, however, at the prospect of a life "watching soaps" as housewife and mother. I asked her how she convinced the others inside to go to law school, and had to chuckle when she replied with her characteristic decisiveness, "I just went and got an application and applied. I was not going to stand for that." In spite of the three children she already had when she began law school and an unsupportive husband, she showed her excellence as law student and lawyer.

The Smart One expresses the advantages she sees in having separate parts of the mind who specialize in their respective jobs as she does in hers. She was created to be pure intellect, speed, and efficiency so that she could satisfy Samantha's father's outrageous intellectual demands during childhood, avoid the torture that followed his dissatisfaction, and not feel the terror that would otherwise have accompanied all learning at home. She is "in charge of anything that requires intelligence," as she told us in Chapter 1. The Smart One therefore has no emotions and feels no empathy or affection. One might think that these attributes would make her work as a lawyer free from the distractions of family ties. This may have been the case when the boundaries between Samantha's parts were more solid. Now, other parts of Samantha's mind are watching and listening inside, including

Samantha. Their background talk distracts The Smart One from the complete concentration she might otherwise achieve. The other parts understand the need to earn a living, but they are not interested in law and exert a pull toward the children's needs familiar to countless guilt-ridden mothers who also work outside the home.

Unlike The Smart One, Samantha's child parts have feelings associated with childhood abuse and are stuck in their state of traumatized responses. When an opposing, screaming lawyer in court sounds like Samantha's father, they have attacks of panic, making it difficult or impossible for The Smart One to stay in control of the body. Some child parts did once gain control and consequently had a panic attack in court, causing The Smart One such embarrassment that she took a leave of absence from her law firm.[2]

Sometimes other parts seem to become simply bored with having to be in the background because of The Smart One's work. Naturally, they sometimes "watch," or "try to participate," or "make comments," and their distractions tire The Smart One and Julia just as such interferences from surrounding people would affect anyone trying to concentrate. The Smart One describes an internal situation much like a family: if one family member takes more time, others feel neglected or unimportant. She is aware of this and seems to understand others' feelings about her work, but she has to ignore their needs: her work comes first. The Smart One makes it clear that she is determined to be a conscientious lawyer in spite of the needs of other parts. "I can't be fussing with them and trying to make them feel better about whether they're important or not when I've got work to do." When she cuts back on clients because of time constraints, she does so in order to retain her standards as a lawyer. "I'm not going to take a client that I can't do a good job with."

Because the Smart One always does the legal work with Julia, who is "nice to people," her character remains consistent. The Smart One's perception that colleagues, employers, and clients have never suspected dual identities is entirely plausible. When Julia is involved, her clients simply think that she is a different aspect of The Smart One's personality and are perhaps grateful for a lawyer who can provide empathy when appropriate, yet be so thoroughly concentrated and businesslike.

The Smart One has never told a colleague or employer the truth about herself. When I asked her what she thought would happen if she told someone, her immediate reply was, "I'd lose my job." Like Gabbi's and Reba's ideals, The Smart One's ideal disclosure reaction would be understanding and the realization that the quality of her work was not affected, but she immediately dismissed the idea of such a response as utopia: "That would never happen." When asked if there was anything she would like a person to say or do in response to a disclosure, I again chuckled at her typically abrupt reply, "Not hit the floor; that would be nice."

Contrasting Two Parts of One Mind

Samantha's experiences of the workday and her attitude toward work outside the home are understandably quite different from The Smart One's. When the topic of her profession was touched on in a general way during the interview, Samantha was the part who replied to my questions; therefore I have both Samantha's and The Smart One's views on some topics concerning work. Eight short sections of the interview reveal the difference between two parts of one mind on the subject of work and career goals. Table 5.1 shows work-related situations from both Samantha's and the Smart One's points of view.

Samantha's experiences of the workday are perhaps analogous to those of someone who is going along for the ride with a friend who has tightly scheduled professional obligations. Only Samantha's experiences are at times more troubled than that and unique to a mind that to outward appearances is an integrated whole but actually composed of sometimes opposing parts. The Smart One's speed and efficiency are essential to the functioning of a lawyer with a large family but at times distressing to Samantha, who fears for her sanity. A therapist eventually explained to Samantha that her description of being "on remote control and somebody else was driving the con-

Table 5.1

---

1. GETTING READY FOR WORK

The Smart One	Samantha
[When I had law offices outside the home,] the initial morning routine was getting the children up and getting them off to school. Then I would pick up my childcare provider and drop her off at the house [to be] with the youngest. [I'm involved in these tasks] if we've gotten in a position where everything's running late and everything has to be done very quickly and organized. Then I'll take over and I'll get it done.	I couldn't keep track of where I was or what I was doing or what I was supposed to do next. It felt like I was on remote control and somebody else was driving the controls and I was going really, really fast—and everything was somehow getting done, but it was just all out of control.

---

2. AT THE OFFICE

The Smart One	Samantha
[Sometimes during the workday] there'd be something going on at school for one of the kids, and some of them [inside] would want to go to that, and I would need to be staying at work to do the work. So we'd have arguments over where we were going to go and what we were going to do next. So that got complicated. Or one of the kids would need a doctor's appointment and there wasn't time to fit it in, and that would cause trouble.	I did really well at law school and got a good job at a fancy law firm. [But] I felt like I wasn't there the whole day, like I didn't know what had happened all day. All day I'd be trying to think about what I needed to do to take care of the kids at home, and I'd be anxious to get out of there so I could go take care of the stuff I needed to do at home. It would be like my head was constantly fighting with itself about what I should be doing and whether I should be doing law work, or going home, or running out to the store to buy something that the kids needed: I was going crazy.

---

3. DOING LEGAL WORK

THE SMART ONE	SAMANTHA
I do all the legal work: . . . deciding what needs to be done for the client; putting together the paperwork; telling the client what needs to be done; going to court; talking to other attorneys on the phone.	[In my law office while the law work was being done] I was looking at this really pretty tree out my window, and I was thinking how neat this was and how cool it was. And I was going into [my second husband's] office and giving him hugs—and daydreaming.

---

4. FUTURE CAREER PLANS

THE SMART ONE	SAMANTHA
I'm unhappy with the legal career now. It's very isolated and very back-stabbing, and it's just not what I thought it would be. I'd like to go to medical school [and] I'm trying to talk them into going. I've always wanted to go to medical school, but I didn't think I could do the math to take the prerequisites because math is not my strong point. But I'm just feeling like maybe if I really worked at it, I could do the math now. [The others don't like this idea very much.] They're tired of my being in school. It takes a lot of time and energy, and they don't get to do as many things as they'd like to do when I'm in school.	I don't know [what my professional goals are except that] I don't think I could go back to a major law firm again, not while I still had kids in the house to raise. So I'm not going to look for that at all. But I'd like to be more financially secure, so I'd like to be working.

trols" was quite accurate: The Smart One was at the wheel. On calmer days, when Samantha and her second husband were both lawyers for the same firm, Samantha would enjoy gazing out the window, having nothing to do with the law work her body and another part were achieving. Gazing out the window or being completely unconscious even while she knows that somehow the work is being done is an experience that does not frighten Samantha because it has been familiar since childhood whenever intellectual demands were made on her. Samantha's sole activity at her office is related to affection, an attribute The Smart One does not need: Samantha goes into her second husband's office and gives him a hug.

When talking about her future career plans, The Smart One has a definite wish, and this time she consults about medical school with other parts who balk at the idea of having the body tied down for such long periods to more learning in which they play no part and have no interest. When I asked Samantha about her future career plans, she did not mention the possibility of medical school, nor did she indicate feeling pulled in different directions concerning her future career. Samantha replied that she wants to continue as a lawyer but only for the financial security, understandable for someone who herself is not involved in the legal profession.

Several of my interview questions reveal my initial, false assumption that my interviewee would be the original identity and that this identity would be the one who works outside the home. For example, one of the questions for which I had to apologize to The Smart One was, "Do you think that you could work outside the home without having parts?" The Smart One responded by simply saying, "No, because I wouldn't be there," confirming in those six words that she understood my misguided question and that she knows she is one part of a person's mind with a specific job to perform. I had also assumed that having a part other than the original identity take control at the workplace would be detrimental to a woman's job performance. Both assumptions were, in Samantha's case, decidedly wrong. Unlike Gabbi or Reba, threats to Samantha's job security come not when another part takes control at work but when the wrong part, including the original identity called Samantha, takes control.

COMMON ASSUMPTIONS, COMPLEX REALITIES

Gabbi, Reba, Samantha, and my other interviewees Barbara and Lucy, therapists; Elizabeth, a teacher; Caroline, an accountant; and Ellie, a retail manager, taught me that common assumptions about parts at the workplace are misguided and that simple conclusions are impossible.

Some people assume for example, that having parts precludes any serious career and is effectively a lifetime disability. Although this was not one of my own assumptions, I began the interviews believing that having parts in itself would be detrimental at work. My interviewees illustrate that the opposite can be true: having parts can enable formerly traumatized women to function by enclosing intolerable feelings and memories, keeping parts of the mind free for learning and concentration so that they perhaps function at higher levels than would normally have been possible. The breakdown of such enclosures can lead to difficulties at work even if the breakdown is the desired result of therapy. Caroline flatly states that having a mind in parts makes it "a lot easier to get things done: one of us does the work and isn't bothered by other things," and Samantha explicitly credits her achievements to her inner specialization. Other professionals' experiences support this positive view.[3] Gabbi, still troubled by lack of communication with other parts of her mind, does find them detrimental at work because they are incapable, unrestrained, and have not yet learned to cooperate with Gabbi. Nonetheless, Gabbi functions competently at a managerial level in her field.

Having assumed that a person's original identity would be the worker, I had concluded that other parts would always be detrimental at the workplace. It seemed counterintuitive to think that dissociated parts, aspects of a "disorder," could take on mature roles essential to a person's profession. Yet, Samantha, Barbara, and Caroline prove exactly this. Each of them has a part who evolved later than the host for all intellectual demands or strictly for work outside the home. Samantha's The Smart One is the most separate of all three because she is responsible not only for work but for all intellectual activity so that unlike Barbara and Caroline, Samantha herself was not trained for her profession. Barbara and Caroline know their work but need a separate set of characteristics to carry it out properly. These characteristics are a one-track mind (literally), maturity, lack of emotion, and for Caroline, self-confidence and a more outgoing personality.

A characteristic of working parts in general is a lack of emotion and of the need for any activities not related to work, making a woman with such a part potentially a more efficient worker than her colleagues with unified minds. The Smart One spoke out in defense of inner specialization when she maintained that with work-related parts on hand, "you always have the right person doing the right job." She herself, as the "right person," tries her best to do her job unobstructed by others inside. Barbara describes her Working Girl as formerly knowing only work, taking no time to eat, chat, or do anything personal or distracting. Only now, after years of therapy, does Barbara occasionally allow herself to relax at work and to incorporate more of her whole self into her job. As an accountant, Caroline has a part called The Working Woman whose sole interest in life is tax returns. Now that therapy has enabled The Working Woman to become less separate from the rest of Caroline's life, Caroline misses the complete concentration she was once able to achieve at work.

Having been corrected about who was the worker, I still surmised that other parts would be either peripheral or troublesome at work, whether a worker part was present or not. Here again, I was mistaken. A part can be the worker and find some parts helpful and others disconcerting. The Smart One welcomes Julia at work but not the other parts of Samantha's mind. Moreover, Barbara, Lucy, and Elizabeth attribute their ability to work exceptionally long hours and override fatigue to having their minds in parts.[4]

Even when the person's first identity is the worker, some other parts of all ages can be useful rather than detrimental at the workplace. The presence of an internal benevolent adult can help the worker part(s) on the job. My interviewees' adult parts appear to generally avoid confusing past and present, and they view the world with the experience of age. Reba made it clear that her adult parts Helper and Circle are essential as child-minders while she works and also help Reba stay calm and efficient when work threatens to overwhelm her. One of Ellie's parts, called Edna, has always been older than Ellie and serves as her voice of wisdom, a kind of inner mother who helps Ellie make wise decisions at home and at work. As a retail manager, Ellie has found that Edna helps her always be calm and polite with customers and to see them as people with wishes and needs, not as things called "customers." Reba and Ellie have both experienced the merging or quiescence of many parts, but their wise adults are still separate within them and still appreciated.

When work involves the care of children or adolescents, child parts receive praise as well. Barbara and Lucy, both therapists who specialize in treating adolescents, and Elizabeth, who teaches special education, told me that having child and adolescent parts helps them understand the needs and wishes of their clients and students so that they can more effectively communicate with them. For these women, when younger parts interfere rather than help at the workplace, they are reacting to long hours without any respite or fun as well as to reminders of past abuse. Other people have observed that child parts who can be useful at work benefit from such contributions to normal daily life.[5]

Nonetheless, in spite of the positive aspects of having parts for some professionals, many nonworking parts are actual or potential disruptions and embarrassments at work, as my interviewees' and others' experiences have shown.[6] Work is smoothest for people in general when emotions, painful memories, or conflicting family obligations do not cloud the mind. So it is with those who have minds in dissociated parts, but for them the problem is magnified by the intensity of emotions, the traumatic nature of memories, and the urgent appeal of inner voices toward family obligations. Some parts' jobs are to keep the working part(s) of the mind unclouded by such memories and emotions. Therefore, some work-related problems are not caused by having parts, but by having non-working parts' memories enter the working part(s) of the mind. For my interviewees, the most common problems caused by nonworking parts were occasional amnesia for workplace events and distractions by inner voices. During the most volatile times, the majority of them found their work interrupted for hours, days, or weeks, often by hospitalizations related to self-injury, suicidal thoughts, or suicide attempts. Half of my interviewees had been hospitalized, three of them several times. Such volatility was sometimes the result of therapy-related leakage of traumatic information previously held intact by non-working parts.

Even during relatively quiet times, the fear of becoming dysfunctional and losing a job always may be present, as it is with Gabbi. A job can offer financial stability, respite from personal problems, and a sense of accomplishment and self-esteem. Work and the workplace are the stabilizing centers of many people's lives and part of their identities. Workers who have parts are no exception, and they dread the thought of losing such an emotionally and financially crucial force. Those who are themselves professional caregivers may also fear failing their own patients or be disquieted by transient urges to abuse the adolescent clients in their care.[7]

Instead of common assumptions and simple conclusions, the effects of having parts on women's work vary according to each woman's system of parts, degree of inner communication and cooperation, and intensity of therapy and workplace stresses. For example, Gabbi's problems at work are greater and more frequent than those of my other interviewees because she is challenged in all three aspects: her system of parts provides no adult helper for her, the host/worker; three of the four young parts who most often take control mainly seem to cause problems; she cannot communicate with the other parts; and workplace stress makes her feel helpless, a feeling dangerously reminiscent of childhood. Gabbi's consciousness alone must try to keep young parts in check and cope with all of life's decisions and workplace stresses. In contrast, all seven other women had at least one helpful adult part each, and the same ratio had reached a workable degree of inner communication and cooperation. All seven also have some other factor that aids their ability to function at work most of the time: either a worker part and/or an internal organizer is present, and/or workplace stress stays within tolerable bounds.

Many of my interviewees find it important to keep the physical and emotional demands of their jobs within limits so that they can work well and take care of themselves. Gabbi, Reba, Samantha, and Barbara have all had to leave jobs that were so stressful they could not maintain functioning. When job stress coincides with any other stress, such as that of recovering memories during therapy, the need to keep workplace stress within limits is even greater. Also important is keeping the workplace as free as possible of emotions and memories similar to past abuse, taking Samantha's screaming opposing lawyer and her panicked young parts as an example. This idea would seem to be contradicted by Barbara and Lucy, both of whom have chosen professions that entail helping adolescents, many of whom have been abused, and by Reba, whose job as a nurse in obstetrics and gynecology puts her in daily contact with procedures some parts of her mind interpret as sexual abuse. However, these three women generally manage to avoid the crucial danger signals of feeling helpless, trapped, or overwhelmed. They are self-confident as workers and have achieved a sense of control over their workplace situations.

SECRECY AND DISCLOSURE

All eight women together illustrate important points about secrecy, stigma, and disclosure. To my interviewees' knowledge, except for intentional disclosures, none of their supervisors or colleagues suspects that these women have dissociated parts of the mind. Even Gabbi's supervisor suspected substance abuse, not parts, when Gabbi behaved markedly inappropriately at a meeting. The one exception is Barbara, a therapist, who let a child part become noticeable in front of a trusted colleague well-versed in dissociated identities, who then suspected the truth.

It surprised me that the therapists Barbara and Lucy had generally positive or neutral responses to disclosures. When Barbara disclosed to a colleague already suspicious of the truth, the colleague recognized a professional advantage in Barbara's personal experience with parts: "That's probably why you're so good with clients who have DID," she said. Lucy is unique among my interviewees in that she has coauthored a self-help book for people who have parts in which she discloses the truth about herself. Among her clients and individual colleagues who have read the book, she has experienced no negative repercussions. Some members of the board of directors of the agency she was running were not pleased, but Lucy was unabashed: "I told them that if I got fired there'd be an APA lawsuit," she said, referring to the American Psychological Association's ability to enforce the law against discrimination at the workplace. Lucy also occasionally verbally discloses to clients who have parts if she thinks disclosure would help in therapy. "Mostly it's a way to get them to realize they're not crazy and not alone," she says.

Ellie's disclosure received a quite different response. She once disclosed to a supervisor during a crisis when memories were returning and parts were turbulent. The supervisor was also Ellie's friend whom Ellie mistakenly thought she could trust with a disclosure told in confidence. To Ellie's dismay, news of her diagnosis spread among colleagues and employers. Many women's fears became reality for Ellie: she found herself the subject of jokes and teasing and realized that although she did not lose her job, knowledge of her diagnosis had forever changed the way her supervisors and colleagues saw her and canceled the possibility of advancement within her company.

All eight women give the strong impression of being dedicated, reliable, ethical workers who invite trust. Nonetheless, almost all of them assume that disclosure would change colleagues' and employers' attitudes toward them and possibly or definitely cost them their jobs. Caroline did lose her job at an accounting office when an employer found out her diagnosis, as she describes in Chapter 6. Yet, women who have parts hold some of the most responsible positions in the workplace, including positions requiring life-or-death decisions such as physicians, therapists, and nurses. My interviewees' descriptions of their working lives suggest that clients or patients will not suffer from this fact.

POINTS TO KEEP IN MIND

- Three factors help smooth workplace functioning:

  - The system of parts provides an adult helper and/or a strong part specializing in work.

  - A high degree of inner communication, negotiation, and cooperation exists among working and nonworking parts.

  - Workplace and/or therapy-related stresses are under control.

- Although a part specializing in work can be an asset, the person as a whole may suffer physical and social deprivation from the workaholic nature of the worker part.

- The feelings associated with workplace stress can be identical to feelings associated with traumatic experiences and cause untimely switching.

- Parts who hold traumatic memories and feelings can be detrimental at work. Yet, without such a separation, more people severely abused as children would be disabled unless skilled therapy had sufficiently lightened the burden of trauma.

6

CAROLINE AT WORK

◉

Caroline is a fifty-seven-year-old married mother of six and grandmother of ten. The following pages, in Caroline's own words, are devoted to Caroline's profession as a self-employed accountant. During the interview, Caroline, as the host, explained that her work as an accountant is done by a part called The Working Woman. During our several meetings for the interview, Caroline once said, "We're basically all one now." Caroline's growing sense of unity is reflected in her speech. She alternately refers to herself and to other parts of her mind as "I" and "she," or as "I" and "we." In the sections where toys are mentioned, some of Caroline's vocabulary seems to still hint at the youthful parts of her mind.

In the course of this chapter, Caroline mentions a few of her parts, including The Mother whom she cannot remember well. All other parts she refers to are also female and of indeterminate age, introduced here in her own words:

- Jessica was never involved with anything sexual, [but] Pam and Jessica are together: [one] actually experienced the abuse; [the other] knows about it.

- Pam was the one that was abused by the father in the house where we lived.

- Terry likes sex; sucks up to people; gets people to love you.

- Vicki didn't have parents. She never lived in the house. She [was] the outside kid, the kid that had fun. As soon as we went out the door, she was the one that took over.

Caroline begins by describing the circumstances in which The Working Woman first appeared. As Caroline continues to talk about The Working Woman, her attitude toward the working part of her mind unfolds.

THE ARRIVAL OF THE WORKING WOMAN

"The last person that we ever split off with was The Working Woman. [Before that,] The Mother was working 'cause she didn't have to interact with anybody: I came into work, sat in a corner, and checked tax returns for math and theory errors, and then I went home. I could make my own hours, I didn't have to be there nine to five, 'cause Charles was still small at the time, so it worked out okay. So for a couple of years we just sat in the corner and did the adding machine, wrote notes to people.

"[Then one day our boss] told [us] that we had to actually do tax returns with people and take on that responsibility and that interaction with other people. So we had to find a way to tell him that we couldn't do it. So we're in this office thinking every day, 'How are we going to get out of this? We need to get out of this because we're not going to be able to do it.'

"And one day, Margaret had six clients in [the office] down the street. So David said to me, 'Margaret needs a hand. There's people waiting down there to have their taxes done.' And I said, 'Oh, okay, I'll go down in a minute.' So finally, after stalling for fifteen, twenty minutes, he said, 'Are you going to go down there? Margaret needs you, she's in a panic.' I said, 'Okay.' So we walked down the street. It was like walking a plank, cement feet; it was the most terrible thing that we remember going through this late in life. It was so difficult that we knew that something was going to happen. It was a buildup of terror, just the same as when you split off because of some trauma. You recognize this feeling, it's just that you're not going to be alone too much longer; you're going to have help. And so the whole walk down there, it was like we knew that this was going to happen. Plus it was the dread of 'What if it doesn't happen? Then we're stuck here.' So it was a whole combination of everything.

"It was awesome when it happened. We're walking down the street and we walked in the door, went directly past all these people, didn't even look at them, went to the back of the building and just stood there and said, 'Okay, we need help.' Then this person came, and she went out and said, 'Who is next? Can I help you?' And we sat down [and] did four tax returns. By then Margaret was done with the other [client], and that was it. That was it. And I remember [thinking], 'This is no problem; [this is] what we do.' So we kept working full-time.

"Afterward, several people that we worked with commented, 'What happened to you?' because it was such a change from somebody that would sit there and not say anything, just say 'Hi' or 'See you tomorrow,' to the outgoing Working Woman. It was really interesting. When it happened and in the days following, we had all this control, like, 'What was the problem for the other person?' And we just continued on like that."

The Working Woman's Characteristics

"The biggest change is between The Working Woman and the rest of us because the rest of us are more together and she's more by herself. But I don't know if you would notice a difference. I think she's like us, outgoing and regular. She knows a lot more about taxes than we do—that makes sense, because she doesn't have anything else to think about. It's pretty cool.

"The Working Woman wasn't involved in things that happened at home. What happened at work was her life—that was it. And there wasn't any interaction between what she did and whatever was going on with kids or anything else; that was taken over by another person when she left work. It was like a totally split day, just like two different people, you know? All

she was interested in was taxes and working. It's always been like that: The
Working Woman just concentrates on the work. She can tell you anything
about her clients, but she really can't tell you that much about the family.
Now it's getting a little bit better, but before [she] wasn't part of it. She can
hear [us talking] now, but she's not interested."

The Advantages of Having The Working Woman at the Job

"If I'm working, all I need to know about is tax laws and my clients. It's a
lot easier than thinking, 'What am I going to have for supper,' or 'It's Steve's
birthday coming up,' or anything outside the box—the box is taxes. We
jump into the box and that's it. We don't need to be knowing all this other
stuff because other people can take care of that. So even though we're more
together [now], this is the way it works best. It works best 'cause I don't
need to be having a bad day because somebody had a fight with the husband or something like that, you see? And my temperament is even all the
time; I just go with the flow because it's about taxes and my clients, and
that's it. So, if the kids are fighting, or my daughter's having a hard time
with her kids, we don't need to know that. And it's worked excellent, really,
it's a much better—I don't know how other people can do it. I don't have
a clue how you can concentrate on your job if you've got fifty million [other]
things going on and you don't have fifty million people [inside] to take care
of them, you know? It must be really difficult. I don't want to do that. So
integration, I'm not going to do that. We can't do it; that would be too confusing to me. Why would you want to?

"I know about [my clients'] lives. That's probably why we have so many
clients, because we remember so much about them. They're like our family, you know what I mean? We see them once a year, [but] if someone
comes in and you [ask], 'How did the wedding go?' 'How's your mother-
in-law doing?' just things that they might have said in passing. And they're,
'Oh, it was fine.' And it kind of makes people feel important—which they

are; they are important to me. But it's just like that's all I have to remember, so that's cool.

"When people call on the phone, they'll say, 'The IRS mailed me a letter. They said there was a problem, and they're giving me $500 less.' Then, immediately everything from their tax return comes into my head. I'll say, 'I bet one of your estimated payments didn't get credited, and maybe you really didn't send it. So you might want to dig up your checks, make sure that you did send in the four payments. 'Cause weren't you supposed to get back $2,100?' So everything is just there in front of my face.

"Some of my clients [say,] 'How do you remember these things?' 'cause I could probably remember their social security numbers as soon as they walk in the door, because that's all I need to know. I see them, [and] everything floods back that I know about them. That's just how it is. It's wild. And you're doing like five hundred people, how do you remember all these things about five hundred people? And they go, 'How do you do that?' So it's amazing, but it's cool. Yeah.

"I think [it's] because that's all we need to know, and when we study taxes, we need to know the theory and all the rules. I'm not bogged down with geography and history and food shopping or anything else, you see? So my whole brain can just focus in on that detail. So I can just look at something that somebody's done before and say, 'There's a mistake there,' and that's how I get a lot of my clients. I probably picked up at least 150 clients by doing that. Because if you bring it in from last year, I look at it and say, 'Wait, this isn't right; this doesn't make sense to me.' I'll do one person's tax return and find something, and then before you know it I have the sister, the brother, and the nephew for clients. So it's more focused, I guess. You're not interrupted with other thoughts—[and] I know my tax laws probably better than anybody else, so that helps.

"If someone calls me and asks me a question, the answer is right there. And there's not too much interference from anyone else because they don't really have that ability. It's always been like [that with] a client, nobody else jumps in and wants to be friends with these people or anything like that. Like Terry, for instance, who likes sex stuff, there's never been any jumping in with a male client, you know what I mean? All that's off limits. It's always a professional but a caring kind of relationship with people. Vicki will come out if people bring their kids. But when she's out, mostly people think that you're just being goofy, and it doesn't last that long.

"I have tons of stamina at work because we separate [from the other parts] great in January. [But] this is June, and I've been really depressed the last month, so I've been staying in bed like till ten o'clock in the morning. It's awful. But during tax season, as soon as it starts, I book my first clients eight o'clock if they need to, and I'm up at six-thirty, and I'll go until nine or ten at night. Because that's all our focus is at that point. I do nothing else. I don't do food shopping, and everybody takes over for me in the house. Like my husband and the kids will be running to the store. I'll take a break and go to therapy, but that's it."

LIVING WITH PARTS TEACHES CAROLINE HOW TO TREAT HER EMPLOYEES

"I was in charge of [one] office for about five years. By keeping the people that I had, and keeping them happy, and treating them decently, my office grew. When I took it over, it was like a 40 thousand dollar office. When I left there it was about 140 thousand. Now we've got people coming back and asking for us, so we built that clientele. I think if you treat people fine then it's a better working relationship. And I think that probably comes a lot from inside, too; it's what we need to do with ourselves. The different personalities working together inside [have] probably got a lot to do with how I work with people outside. Because you learn that. My biggest thing is that you want to treat people the way you want to be treated yourself. That's just how I am. But I think a lot of that came with learning how to manage all of us.

"I think [I manage inside by] being kind; just not saying, 'Well, this is the way it's going to be; these are my rules and we're sticking by them.' You need to have a lot of negotiation inside and take other people's feelings into account. Like, I can't just say, 'I'm here until April fifteenth and tough cookies. You can come back after that. That's the way it is.' I mean, it's not fair to anybody else inside that they can't do what they want to do, [that] Vicki doesn't get to play with anything.

"It's just something that we learned 'cause when the walls [between us] came down we started knowing about each other inside and what we're all about. Then you had to learn to live with that. And sometimes that person wasn't a very nice person, maybe not up to my standards of being an upstanding citizen. But you need to learn why they were like that, what it was that led them to do these things. So I think it's just that we pay attention to other people, really pay attention to them. [I think that's] got a lot to do with it, although I don't think anybody inside is a nasty kind of person. We're just not like that. So maybe, in general, we're basically kind of nice.

WHEN NONWORKING PARTS INTERFERE

"When we were so unsettled, [it used to be that even during the tax season] there was a lot of turmoil inside because no one else was getting any time. It upset people if they didn't have as much time as they needed. Especially when we were doing journaling [for] therapy, we wanted to just be writing, writing, writing. And it was always an interruption that we would need to work because we felt like we should be focusing on ourself, just going to therapy and working on that. So those few years with Paul, the first therapist, were hard for us for being able to work, especially when everyone was coming out. There was so much traffic of people that wanted their time, that wanted their therapy. They wanted to be concentrated on *them*: 'This is *my* time.'

"So when we had the office in a building, we made rules: they would get to have all their time before we got there, and then, at the top of the escalator, I would come out, and then it was my time. They couldn't come back until we were leaving [and] it was time to go down the escalator. Then that was their time again. That worked out pretty well. That was a rule—Vicki has a lot of rules; she's the rule keeper. That just became something that happened. And as it happened more and more, they really didn't need even that time, you know what I mean? It didn't have to be every day as long as they knew they could have it.

"[And we have had times when a child part has appeared at work.] Vicki actually had a fight with a little kid—oh God! The little boy was there with his mother, [my coworker's] client. [The boy] brought in a Burger King toy, and I think it must have been a toy that we never saw before. So he was playing with the Burger King toy on the desk. We were doing taxes for somebody and suddenly it was like, 'What's that toy?' And the little boy was like, 'It's *my* toy.' So it's like, 'I know it's your toy, just what is it? Can I see it?' Then he was like, 'No, it's *my* toy.' [But] she really wanted to see the toy, so she got up and went over—and I'm going, 'Oh, jeez.' And that year we had all these other toys that we'd brought in, little Mighty Macs [that] come in a clam shell and you open it up and inside there's scenes, and they might have dinosaurs in there—it was wicked cool. And so I said to this little kid, 'Want to see these toys? These are wicked cool. Do you know about Mighty Mac stuff?' He said, 'I don't care about Mighty Mac; this is my toy.' And I says, 'Well, you can at least share it. I just want to see it. I'm not going to take it home.' And he wouldn't share it with me. I said, 'You're a jerk!' And his mother looked at me, but I didn't care. [Later, my coworker] said, 'I thought you were going to come and grab it out of that kid's hand. I was getting a little scared there.' But we did go to Burger King on the way home, just so I could get one of those for myself. [She laughs.] That's not fair. Some kids are really stupid, you know?

"We used to bring our Mighty Mac stuff into that office 'cause Paul, [my therapist,] said that can be a rule: you can bring in your toys to work. And so we brought them in [and] kept them there all in a bag. The excuse was that little kids come with their parents to do tax returns, and so the kids could play with my toys while they're there, 'cause I share really good. So everybody knew that we had toys there, but they just thought it was 'cause of that. They didn't know the real reason.

"[One time] we had a therapy appointment for Saturday afternoon, but I was working Saturday. So I was going to have to leave work and go up there. So I got this one client and I was doing her tax return, and she was kind of flighty, she really didn't know her information. What happened is, it wasn't me that was doing her taxes. It was somebody else, whoever was going to go up and see Paul, probably Pam or Jessica. We were in a hurry to get her out of there so we could leave, so we kind of rushed her through it. The next year, she came back. I was doing her tax return, and she said, 'I almost didn't come back this year.' And I said, 'Oh, how come?' And she said, 'The person that I had last year was so rude to me, so rude.' And I says, 'Jeez, everybody's really nice in this office; I'm surprised that you would perceive someone as rude that worked here.' So I pulled out last year's tax return, and I'm looking at it, and it was my signature on the bottom. And I said, 'Gee, *I* did your tax return last year.' And she says, 'No, no, no, it wasn't you that did it; you're very nice. The person that did it last year was very rude to me.' So I looked at the date on it, and I remembered that what had happened was that we were in a hurry to get to Paul; it was a crucial time in our therapy. And probably she just got shoved under, poor thing. So I says, 'I'm so sorry.' She says, 'Oh, don't worry about it. You're very nice, dear.' She just didn't want to hear it. 'Whoever did it last year, I don't like her,' she said. And I says, 'Oh, okay.' I couldn't convince her that it was me that did it—because, actually, it wasn't."

Seasonal Conflicts Among Parts: From April Sixteenth to January First

"If this was a fifty-two-week-a-year job, I really don't know if we could do [it] as good. Because we do taxes, we just need to focus for fourteen weeks out of the year, until April fifteenth. And so for all the others to give up time for one person to do the job is okay, because they know we have the whole rest of the year to do things, and we don't need to be that focused all the time.

"As soon as tax season is over, I really don't function very well in the working capacity. It's over, but I still have a few things left to do—and it just keeps getting postponed. I'll get behind and won't do things I'm supposed to do. And you can get in trouble like that. I'm being sabotaged by others that say, 'You've had enough time; forget this.' You know what I mean? I sit down at the computer, and all of a sudden a game comes on and we sit there for hours playing a stupid game when I have work to do. I lose a lot of time like that, and then the work never gets done. I get pushed out of the way. That's actually what therapy was about last week. It was, 'Yeah, we need time here.'

"It's wicked frustrating, and it comes from different levels. I'm frustrated because I can't get to the work; other people are frustrated because I'm doing work instead of doing what they want to do. [They let me know that] by taking the time and not letting me get to that level to do the work. It's like I have no real control over it. It's not just a reluctance. How can I describe it? I think if you're a regular person you just put stuff off if you're feeling like, 'I'll do this later.' I don't know; I have no point of reference for that. I just know that I lose time, and I'll lose the whole thing. I just found the note yesterday that one poor guy called me and asked me for a copy of his tax return and to look something up. He's selling his house, and he wanted to know what the consequences would be. Apparently we took down all the information that we needed and must have said we were going to call him right back. That was about a month ago. When I saw the note yesterday when I was cleaning off my desk, it was the first time I was looking at it. I was saying, 'What the hell?' And then it comes to me that I remember talking to him. I says, 'Oh shit!' I think I've probably lost a few clients that got really ticked off at me 'cause I didn't return phone calls. You feel like such a jerk that you didn't follow through on this.

"And I find my messages—like, once you listen to my messages on my machine, they go into another place, so if [one of my parts] has already heard them, [and] I come in and press the button for new messages, they won't show there. You see what I mean? So I've gone in the place where listened-to messages go and heard people calling back two, three, and four times for stuff, and I don't remember! I never listened to the messages, somebody else did inside of me. It's like other people totally take over. So I don't have a handle on being able to do a good job at this time of the year. They still want the time for themselves and for other things that are going on. We're getting better at cooperation, it used to be a lot worse. But it's still there. In January, that all goes away and it's totally work."

CAROLINE DISCLOSES HER DIAGNOSIS AT WORK

"When I was working for a [tax service firm] in the summertime, they hired Jamie [as] assistant manager. And 'cause we were there all the time, we got friendly and close. At some point, I told her about the MPD.* She understood it and we talked about it, 'cause most of the time it was like a nonissue. But she was aware of it. Then something happened with a client that I had [about] not answering his calls—like I told you how this time of year I don't work very well. He got really mad and complained to [the head office] that he'd given me his stuff and that I didn't give back his taxes early enough. And Claudia, the district manager, called me in. So I went up to the office and Jamie was there. And Claudia said to me, 'Jamie tells me that you're dealing with a lot of personal stuff.' So I said, 'Yeah.' Now, Claudia will be nice as pie to you, but then she'll take the information and stab you in the back. I should have realized it, but she was being nice as pie, and she's like, 'Well, what's going on?' So we told her—big mistake. I was trying to explain to her that that is probably why we didn't get back to this person: once April fifteenth is over, other personalities want their time.

---

*MPD stands for multiple personality disorder, the term formerly used for dissociative identity disorder.

"So, in October, I got a letter saying that I wasn't available for rehire. Let me tell you, this has never been done in the whole history of anything! They'll take the worst people in the world, people who never show up for work, people that you can't rely on. And all these people never get fired. I know that because when I was processing supervisor, I was working on that end of it. And the only thing you could do to get rid of them was not put them on the schedule. But they're available for rehire next year. Nobody's ever gotten a letter, because they need somebody sitting in that seat no matter how bad they are. So I got this letter, and it said that I wasn't available for rehire. I said, 'Oh my God, it's got to be that. There's no other explanation.'

"I think Claudia was scared. Even though she had known me for fifteen years, I think she was probably scared of the effect of whatever perception she had of MPD, probably that I was going to go bonkers in the office, I don't know. I never called her, never spoke to her again. I just said, 'Okay, I guess that settles it. I'll be going into business for myself.' So I bump into a lot of my clients from the tax firm here and there, you know, shopping, whatever. And so whoever I bumped into I said, 'Apparently I'm not going to [the firm]; I'm going to work out of my house.' So it all worked out, it was like this thing that's just meant to be. That's when I started working at home.

"If it happened now, I would probably be strong enough to sue her for discrimination. But that has to be done really fast; [and,] of course, you're not strong enough at the time, and you don't want everybody to know all your business. But [if I had known] that things can be sealed and you can do it as a Jane Doe, I probably would have done it. [But now it's] too late.

"[I've disclosed to colleagues.] Like Jean, for instance, was my friend, and she was a bookkeeper. Once she found out, she said everything made sense. Deborah was another one that said that. Deborah was an office manager, and we got to be very close. Once I told them—which wasn't till probably '95, and they'd known me since the '80s—but once I told them, it's like they weren't surprised. Jean said, 'Now, everything makes sense.' So apparently they see things that I don't. You know what I mean? Like, I think that I'm just regular, but apparently they saw things that I didn't.

"[For example,] Jean said, when she first met me, how timid I was and how I never spoke to her—because it wasn't me. And she says, 'I'd come in and say "Good morning," and you never talked to me or anything. And then, all of a sudden I come back to work in January, and there you are, this take-control kind of person. And I'm going, "That's not the same woman!"' But people don't think of MPD, you know; they just don't connect it.

"If my clients ever found out, I can't imagine that I would lose any from it. Because I tend to associate with people that I think would understand. And probably anybody that I would lose I wouldn't miss anyway. I know there've been a few times when I've had clients that I thought were MPD. And we would have conversations about things, not coming right out, but I would make reference to my website for abuse survivors. I would just mention that we have people that come on there with dissociative disorders and MPD, the different things that can happen to people because of abuse. I would just talk in generalities like that. And then that frees them up. I suspected that they were, only because sometimes you can just tell. It's this thing between people, I don't know what it is. Just some kind of a sixth sense."

POINTS TO KEEP IN MIND

- A buildup of terror reminiscent of childhood abuse can cause a new part to appear in adulthood if the existing parts are not appropriate for the person's needs.

- Nonworking, nondestructive parts need to be allowed to express themselves at negotiated times in appropriate settings. Such self-expression can be crucial to smooth functioning.

- For people with one or more parts of the mind who specialize in work, lack of cooperation by nonworking parts can mean loss of control and amnesia for work.

- A person with parts may try to overcome any negative aspects of non-working parts but keep the advantages of a working part's single-minded concentration.

- Judicious disclosure of the diagnosis to trusted people allows them to make sense of years of puzzling behavior.

- Disclosure can have irrevocably negative consequences if the trusted person does not keep the disclosure confidential or is in a position of power and does not fully understand the meaning of having parts.

7

Experienced Innocence: Adolescent Identities Who Seek Sex

◉

Q. *Samantha, can you tell me why the sexual part of your mind called Cecelia came?*

A. Well, [the intellectual part called] The Smart One was kind of doing all the jobs. And there was a timed test that she had to do on Sunday night for my father. She had to do it in a particular amount of time—and she couldn't do it. And so, Cecelia came to do it.

Q. *What kind of test was that?*

A. We had to satisfy him in a certain number of minutes, whatever he decided.

Q. *Satisfy him?*

A. Make him have an orgasm with our mouth.

Q. *Was this a regular event?*

A. [Every] Sunday night.

Q. So Cecelia did it from then on?
A. Yeah, she took over that whole job.

⊙

Like the forty-two-year-old Samantha, many formerly abused women
continue in adulthood to have one or more parts excluded from their
bodies' sexual activities. When I asked Cecelia how she works out her sexual relationships with Samantha, she replied, "There's nothing to work out.
When I come out, she goes away." Cecelia's entrance cue is anything to do
with sex. Cecelia invariably enters on cue, and Samantha invariably "goes
away." Samantha illustrates that having another part of the mind ready and
willing for sex can leave the host with a body more sexually experienced
than she would like, but with the consciousness of a virgin.

This type of innocence depends on the alternate control of mind and
body provided by parts like Cecelia, whose original job was to protect
Samantha's consciousness from years of incestual abuse. Now, Cecelia comes
out whenever "things are getting more sexually overtoned." This is a logical continuation of her defense of Samantha's consciousness from sex. However, Cecelia also invites sex on her own, rather than simply obeying the
need to take over the mind whenever a situation becomes sexual. The sex-
related parts of four other women I interviewed also used to invite sex or
still do so, and such parts are evidently common among women who have
dissociated identities.[1] In families, an adolescent girl whose main interest
in life is having sex is likely to cause her parents concern and distress. Having such a "girl" as a part of the mind who periodically controls the body
is even more difficult. The girl inside the mind is led not only by "interest"
in sex, she was created for sex and having sex is her job. These formerly
abused parts seem to actively invite sex for a variety of reasons, with sometimes dangerous consequences. I tried to discover why parts of these five
women's minds invite sex and in what ways their behavior affects the person as a whole.

Samantha's Part Cecelia:
"I Don't Like Watching"

Samantha, as the sum of her parts, is a lawyer. In the previous interview excerpt with her, she describes Cecelia's first appearance as the part responsible for sex and for almost all conversations or experiences related to the body. Only childbirth remains as Samantha's conscious body-related experience. After passing the father's "timed test," Cecelia remained as the part specializing in sex. Cecelia introduced the concept of the sex-related identity in Chapter 1, when she told me in her own voice about her job as an adolescent part of Samantha's mind. Samantha was switched to Cecelia as soon as I began asking about the topic of sex, although I was aware of the switch only when Cecelia eventually introduced herself.

According to Samantha, Cecelia seeks sex because she wants it, and she wants it because "that's her job." Cecelia does not care whether she has sex with many or with one as long as she is active. During Samantha's two marriages, Cecelia sought no other men. With Samantha now divorced, dating is not enough to satisfy Cecelia unless it includes having sex. On dates, Cecelia is switched into control whenever things become "sexually overtoned," just as she was during the years of abuse, and she has sex with any man she dates.

Samantha, on the other hand, is a part of the mind whose primary roles are wife and mother. She would like to meet men because she hopes to find someone with whom she can form a stable, permanent relationship. With this goal in mind, she advertises in an Internet dating resource. However, Cecelia has other ideas. When a man responds to the ad, Cecelia writes a provocative e-mail in reply, one that implies by its tone that the respondent can expect sex on the first date, an expectation reinforced by Cecelia's choice of clothing: form-fitting red outfits and see-through tops with no bra. Samantha tells how her attempts to find a life partner are thwarted by Cecelia who automatically appears as soon as a man's speech or behavior imply sex.

We'll meet for dinner and then . . . well, if my kids aren't home, we'll go back to my house. Or sometimes we'll go back to their house, and then Cecelia usually has sex with them. I do [know about this while it's happening] because my therapist set it up that we all know what's going on with everybody. I'm paying attention [by] watching the TV screen. I don't like watching. Then we arrange another time to meet and go home. [And when we meet the second time,] the same thing. There are a couple of them that I like, but I don't know if they like me. I don't know if they're in the relationship just for the sex or if they like me.

Samantha gains her aim of meeting men, then unwittingly behaves in such a way that she never gets to know them. Understandably, at such times she does not appreciate her "TV screen," her newly achieved ability through therapy to remain co-conscious and watch her body when another part of her mind has control.

Cecelia will also do her job to make money. During a personal financial crisis, all parts of Samantha's mind had an internal meeting to discuss possible solutions. At the meeting, Cecelia took the floor, saying, "Hell, I know how to make money; I've done this before," referring to the time during her first marriage when she sold her body to her husband's friends to pay for law school. Drawing on that experience for a financial crisis after her divorce, Cecelia used the Internet to pick up men. For three weeks she made money having sex, leaving her body with genital warts that had to be surgically removed.

CAROLINE'S PART TERRY: "I DIDN'T EVEN KNOW THEIR NAMES"

Caroline, as the sum of her parts, is a fifty-seven-year-old accountant. Terry is a part of Caroline's mind who used to be responsible for taking abusive sex. Caroline was a teenager when Terry first appeared, and Terry has remained a part with adolescent attitudes and behaviors and a liking for sex. The recollection of Terry's sex-seeking years makes Caroline cringe. Terry was, indeed, active, causing years of sexual experiences that Caroline is embarrassed to recount and cannot completely recall.

> Terry's totally teen stuff was all just a game. I don't think I've ever had a relationship with anyone that really meant anything. . . . There were some people that you cringe about as soon as they walk out the door. There were a few times I didn't even know their names, you know what I mean? And then, at some time in my life, people were just calling and coming over, people that I didn't even know. I don't know where that is in my life, [but] I can see it happening.

Because of Terry's "teen stuff," Caroline became pregnant at fifteen and married the baby's father, who immediately joined the navy. She had a second and third baby after each of her husband's two leaves and attracted strangers to her bed in between. Terry continued her activities for years, bringing in more men than Caroline can count, though never receiving money from the men as far as Caroline knows.

Having sex is Terry's way of gaining power over men, the feeling she likes most about sex. Caroline puts it this way:

> It wasn't so much the sexual part of it, it was the control over—I would say over men. It was just like, "I could make you do whatever I want, you jerk," you know what I mean? And it wasn't that she was in love with these people that she was going to bed with or anything like that. It was just getting them to do it and then cutting them out of her life, you know, screw you and leave.

Terry actively and repeatedly sought men until Caroline, as an adult part and host, became able at age thirty-five to be conscious for sex and control her sexual activities. This change occurred for unknown reasons and before Caroline entered therapy. Terry now remains inside for jobs such as business deals, which require feeling in control of men, thus cleverly remaining useful to Caroline in ways more appropriate to her adult needs.

GABBI'S PART HEATHER: "I DIDN'T KNOW HOW I COULD BE PREGNANT"

Gabbi, as the adult host, is a forty-two-year-old director of finance and administration. Two other parts of her mind are adolescents who occasionally take control of consciousness and seek masochistic sex. The part Gabbi mentioned most often is Heather. When Heather occasionally takes control of the body during sex with Gabbi's female partner, Heather is aggressive and also requests pain. Heather is emotionally and cognitively fourteen years old and does not like to eat. She perceives herself as very thin and "fairly attractive," Gabbi says, with Heather's long hair obligingly blond, the color Gabbi's parents wanted for their daughters. Arrayed in her beautiful self-perception, Heather goes in search of men and abusive sex, and Gabbi returns home bruised and bewildered. Referring to Heather's sexual excursions, Gabbi says,

> Probably in college was the first time I remember that I found myself in that situation, after the fact. I don't think I had a total understanding of what that meant—how I got there, how it happened. That was still during the time where I thought I was losing my mind and that there was something drastically wrong, not really understanding and not really wanting to know what that was.

Heather has been actively seeking sex since high school, when she would have one-night stands instead of dates. Gabbi sees this focus on quick sex partly as her way of maintaining distance so that no one would know "what was really me," a distance she now maintains in her professional life. Because of Heather, Gabbi has "woken up" in hotel rooms and backs of cars to find herself with strangers. She usually simply leaves without explanation.

> Some of them [I can remember, but] there was a point in my life that I was pregnant and had no knowledge of anybody I had slept with; I didn't know how I could be pregnant. I had an abortion. I'm not sure what [a] pregnancy would have done to me psychologically, so I think it was the right thing to do. But it's a huge regret, it's a huge loss.

Gabbi now experiences amnesia for sex less frequently, but when it does occur, the last thing Gabbi remembers is feeling particularly pressured, not being able to "take it," needing to escape. Gabbi regains consciousness to find herself lying with a stranger in bed.

Gabbi does not yet know the part Heather very well, and therefore does not know Heather's reasons for actively seeking sex. However, Heather is continuing the function she originally came for, perhaps deliberately making it an action of choice to transform the memory of her helplessness when she was summoned as a child to her sadistic father's bedroom.

Elizabeth's Parts Black Betty and Body Part: "I Remember Being Up on the Ceiling"

Elizabeth, as the host, is an adult, professional part of her mind who is a forty-two-year-old teacher. In Elizabeth's sexual life, two other parts called Black Betty and Body Part seem to have been especially significant during adulthood. Both parts are adolescents, and each has a specific role different from the other. Black Betty used to dress in black, swear, be aggressive, and have sex with numerous men. Black Betty seems to have attracted men to her and to have been active mainly before and between her marriages. Elizabeth describes Black Betty as sexy, provocative, and wild, with a raw way of speaking. Elizabeth's other sex-related identity is called Body Part, whose job was to take her cue from Elizabeth's two husbands and behave however the two men wanted. During one such incident, Elizabeth thought of another name for Body Part.

> This sounds really weird, I know, but my first husband and I had gone away, and the hotel room had mirrors on the ceiling. And I remember being up on the ceiling, but I could see my own reflection—and I saw myself [during sex]. I thought, "God, Performing Bear down there"; I saw myself as a performing bear. It wasn't good.

Here Elizabeth describes depersonalization, with part of her mind observing another part's actions during sex with her husband. The part called Elizabeth was, as usual during marital sex, "up on the ceiling," only this time, the ceiling was covered with mirrors, giving her an unwanted view of her body obeying, like a well-trained animal, all her husband's wishes.

For many years, Elizabeth was usually not present during sex. Sometimes she was completely "gone" and would come back to find herself with men she and a girlfriend had met at a bar. Throughout both of her marriages, Elizabeth "floated" outside her body during sex and watched it with disgust and shame:

> [My body did] anything and everything; more than I choose to share. It was just gross. That was not good to watch [myself] because then I'd have all the feelings of being slutty or being trash, what men told me I was as a child, or feeling dirty and guilty and a bad girl.

Now and then Elizabeth would find a garter or a sexy corset around her house and wonder how they got there and when she had worn them. Her shame about sex was so great that years of therapy passed before she was willing to talk about the topic with her therapist.

BARBARA'S PART SLUT GIRL: "I WASN'T PRESENT"

Barbara, as the sum of her parts, is a social worker. A part of her mind is called Slut Girl, a name that suggests what the rest of Barbara's mind thinks of Slut Girl's demeanor. Envisioned as having jet black hair, Slut Girl came to Barbara's aid during abuse, but not until Barbara was a teenager. Slut Girl took over for younger parts who had endured abuse since infancy. She was sixteen when she first appeared and has remained that same age over the years. Barbara said that Slut Girl originally came to prevent the unendurable humiliation of powerlessness. Slut Girl turned incestual sex into an activity of her choice, transforming powerlessness and helping to spare part of Barbara's mind all memory of those years. When Barbara left home to go to college, Slut Girl continued her job.

> Slut Girl was only focused on sex; she would have sex with everyone. That was just her way. It was like, "This is the one that does sex, and I'll be *her* now." I wasn't present. I *had* to dissociate because anyone who'd asked me, "Do you want to have sex?" I would. Even when I knew that I didn't want to have sex with men, I would still have sex with them. If they asked me, I would just go, "Oh, yeah, whatever," [said in a tone of indifference] which was not good, but fortunately I outgrew that before things got too out of hand.

As Barbara says, Slut Girl used to have sex with anyone who asked. Evidently there was no shortage of men asking. Barbara calls this her "promiscuous period," during which her consciousness as the host had no awareness of having sex. Slut Girl seems to have played a more passive and acquiescent but also inviting role, more like the provocative Black Betty, as compared with the parts Cecelia, Heather, and Terry, who actively seek men and sex.

WHY SEEK REMINDERS OF THE PAST?

The eight women I interviewed experienced childhood abuse comparable in length, type, and familial involvement. During childhood and adolescence, all of them had parts of their minds in charge of taking the sexual abuse. Why, then, do five of these women have parts who invite sex or actively seek it, and others do not? Certainly such differences reflect the uniqueness of outwardly similar experiences, of each person's psychological structure, and consequently the uniqueness of life with parts for each person who has them. However, I found interesting similarities among the women who, as adults, have parts who specialize in seeking sex. These similarities may offer clues as to why some parts invite sex rather than simply continue their jobs of taking over the body when sex does occur.

Among my interviewees, parts who invite sex are adolescents. Some are created during adolescence, but others are created during childhood, with the child's imagination conjuring a girl who has reached sexual maturation and can therefore better "take" the abuse. No matter when they were created, they remain emotionally and cognitively adolescents who see themselves as sexually mature but always young, always willing. Like other parts of the mind, these parts remain active after the childhood abuse has ceased.

Judging by my interviewees, such parts have certain characteristics:

- *They perceive themselves as attractive or sexy.* These parts know how important the perception of physical attraction can be to a woman who wants to be sexually active.

- *They feel young.* Although the body may be middle-aged and post-menopausal, the sexually active parts perceive themselves as being in the smooth and freshly rounded bodies of new maturity.

- *They need to be active.* These parts do not simply endure sex, they have learned to like and need it. One reliable partner may or may not suffice. If monogamy does not offer much sex, or if the sexual partner is the "wrong" sex, or not abusive during sex, the sexual parts of the mind may seek partners elsewhere.

- *They are able to pass as the host.* A part who spoke sexually enticingly in a child's voice from an adult's body or frequently played with toys would not get the reaction she sought from prospective sexual partners. Furthermore, she would give herself away, a dangerous thing to do. In order to pass, the adult body must have an adult's vocal range and a reasonable demeanor and vocabulary. The first people for whom she must pass as "normal" are the original abusers. This is probably one reason why a new adolescent part often first appears when the body has reached adolescence.

The adolescent parts who have these characteristics remain active for a number of reasons, job description being a major one. Like the workforce in the outside world, these parts do not want to lose their jobs, and they need to remain active, to feel useful. A sexually active part's primary duty was to protect other parts from the experience of sexual abuse and/or from its emotional impact. Even if the host wishes to experience consensual sex in adulthood, other parts believe she cannot tolerate it and must be protected. Consequently, the host blacks out, watches from a distance, or is emotionally numb. Gabbi as the adult host, for example, is completely unconscious when her adolescent part Heather is with a man, but even with Gabbi's chosen female partner, the sex Gabbi is able to experience and remember is pure physical sensation, devoid of thought, emotion, or cognizance of the mate. As Gabbi says, "Sex is such a purely physical, unemotional, unintellectual thing for me that it really is irrelevant whether they're male or female, or that it's in a relationship, not in a relationship, love or not love." Nonabusive sex with a female partner is evidently not what the Heather part needs. Sex with a sadistic man is the job she was created for, and she goes out in search of that specific work.

A part may also transform her experiences during adolescence so that she believes the abuse is her choice and that she controls the situation, as Barbara's part Slut Girl did. Once the body has reached adolescence and is ready for procreation, new feelings of physical shame and modesty develop, feelings that were either unknown or less potent as a young child. Perhaps these feelings increase the likelihood that the mind will need to reverse the emotional trauma of helplessness while the body is exposed and humiliated by abuse. A solution is for one or more parts to perceive themselves as wanting the sex and being in control of it. Turning the abuse into an act of her choice protected Barbara against the reality of helplessness. If part of the mind's function was to believe that repeated abusive sex was an activity of choice, logically, in adulthood, that part may continue to make sex a repeatedly sought-after activity.

Similarly, a part may reverse her childhood experiences by becoming the seducer rather than the seduced, the user rather than the used. As Caroline said, feeling "control over men" was Terry's reason for seeking sex. If a child or adolescent became sexually aroused during the abuse, she may need to avenge her helpless, humiliating physical response by repeatedly making men desirous. Among my interviewees, only Samantha reported that she was aware of having received money for sex. However, other studies show that some formerly abused women's parts work as prostitutes, so great is their repeated need to undo their childhood helplessness by playing an active, controlling role.[2] Other research also shows that some women need to reexpress the feelings they had during the original abuse,[3] feelings that only a part of the mind can acknowledge.

Adolescent parts may also simply not realize that they can say no. Where would they have learned that they have the power to refuse? They are acquiescent because they know no other way of behaving unless years of relearning have taught them otherwise. This perceived powerlessness was evidently one of the reasons Slut Girl used to have sex with many men. As Barbara said, "Anyone who'd asked me, 'Do you want to have sex?' I would. Even when I knew that I didn't want to."

BECOMING INVOLVED WITH
ABUSIVE PARTNERS

The pervasive influence of sex-related parts of the mind helps explain why people who have DID so often become involved with abusive partners,[4] like Samantha's first husband or Gabbi's nameless men, especially if they come to their partners straight from abusive homes and with no acknowledgment or understanding of past experiences. Abusiveness may have been the only kind of attention or physical "affection" they knew. Also, a child or adolescent can become sexually aroused during abusive sex and can also learn to associate pain with sexual arousal. Reexperiencing the sensations she learned to want during abuse may be a reason she becomes involved with abusive partners later in life. Conversely, her body may feel chronically numb, so that during physical abuse the blood from cuts, abrasions from ropes, and bruises from beatings are welcome as signs that her body is alive, and perhaps also as signs of the punishment she feels she deserves.

Logically, some women tend to form strong emotional bonds to people like their original abusers on whom they were emotionally and physically dependent.[5] Therefore, in adulthood it may feel natural to a woman to continue in the role of victim to an abusive partner. The sexual adolescent part would not perceive the dangers in her behavior that outside observers—and other parts of her own mind—would perceive. In addition, sex-related adolescent parts may not perceive sadistic sex as abusive. During childhood, in self-protection, the sexual part may neither acknowledge the abuser as a relative nor acknowledge the abuse as a violation. This was true of Samantha and her sexual part Cecelia, who went from abusive parents to an abusive husband. Therefore, possibly no part in control during sex in adulthood has learned to recognize abusive acts as violations.

A child's belief that she is somehow bad and responsible for being abused persists into adulthood. Therefore, punishment through continued abuse seems logical even as an adult. Caroline and the part called Terry are examples. Caroline learned as a child that she would not be allowed to go out and play with her friends until she had gratified her father's desire. Eager to play as a child, Terry would then behave invitingly toward the father to speedily fulfill his requirement and be free. This added fuel to Caroline's firm belief that as a child, she brought on the abuse and is a "whore" and "slut" who deserves degradation. Such beliefs are common among formerly abused women, who may also hear such accusations from the abuser.[6]

However, even without sex-related parts, some of the aftereffects of trauma, such as feeling numb or helpless, can encourage abuse during adulthood. Dissociation may lead to a lack of awareness for potential danger,[7] and helplessness can lead a woman to feel incapable of escaping a situation she recognizes as dangerous. Some formerly abused adults describe becoming unable to move or automatically submissive in the presence of a powerful, threatening, and abusive person.[8] Such immobility in response to stress and threat is a reaction that evolved for survival.[9]

CATALYSTS FOR THE NEGATIVE, PROTECTORS OF THE POSITIVE

Undesired, unprotected, and indiscriminate sex was or still is a fact of life for all five women who have sexually active adolescent parts. In contrast are the three interviewees whose sex-related parts are strictly or mainly passive. For example, Lucy, as the host and social worker, used to remember having sex, but was physically and emotionally "gone" until sex was over. Lucy did not go in search of sex or have an unusual number of partners, although she had reached the age of thirty before she realized, with a therapist's help, that she could refuse the sex another person wanted.

Ellie, as the host and retail manager, knows about a sixteen-year-old part called Myra who came not during childhood, like Ellie's other parts, but during a single traumatic event as a teenager: rape at knifepoint by a gang of men when Ellie was fourteen. Myra does not seek men as a result; she hates them and is sexually attracted to women. In high school, Ellie was once caught looking in an interested way at a classmate who had openly declared herself lesbian. Rumors spread about Ellie's own sexuality. Yet, the Myra part does not actively seek female partners, and the parts of Ellie's mind who took the childhood torture inflicted by groups of adults stopped taking over in adulthood. Interestingly, Ellie has always been able to remember her own father's sexual abuse and is able to remain fully conscious during sex in adulthood.

In contrast to both Ellie and Lucy, Reba, as the host and nurse, has chosen to abjure sex. She does, however, communicate with a thirteen-year-old part called Jen, who "holds our sexuality and wants to date," Reba says. In other words, part of Jen's job is to enclose and preserve Reba's social and sexual instincts, hoping that she will someday be able to incorporate them into her life.

The three women without sexually aggressive parts have had problems related to their sexuality. However, none of them has had the potentially dangerous sexual turbulence caused by such parts. Their sexual actions cause them no distress; they do not feel shamed, denigrated, or physically endangered because of sex in adulthood. In contrast, women with sexually active parts are sometimes called promiscuous by mental-health professionals or use that term themselves for their behavior. *Promiscuous* seems a needlessly pejorative term, given the complex reasons behind these women's sexual actions. Nonetheless, my interviewees show that this same behavior and their formerly protective, sex-seeking parts endanger health and personal safety. Rape, sexually transmitted diseases, physical abuse, unwanted pregnancies, and abortions are some of the possible consequences. Added to these are the chaos of multiple strangers entering the home for sex or of "waking up" in strange places with strange bedfellows. Sex-related parts may also be the catalyst for a teenage pregnancy and marriage, with only part of a woman's mind engaging in such significant involvements.

Sex-related parts have one-track minds, and the sexuality they preserve is often distorted, causing a maze of negative, sometimes devastating consequences. Nonetheless, these parts not only shielded the parts of the mind in charge of daily functioning during childhood or adolescence, but they preserved a willingness to have sex in adulthood. After such abusive childhoods, renouncing sex as an adult for a long while or forever would seem a logical step. I was surprised at how many of the women I spoke with who had endured years of sexual abuse went on to form sexual attachments. In fact, all but one of my interviewees have shown themselves capable of entering nonabusive sexual attachments, though some took years of therapy to achieve. Even Reba, the one exception, who renounced sex as soon as she escaped her parents' power, now considers a sexual attachment a future possibility. Half of the women I spoke with have also found that they, as the adult hosts, can now both experience and control their own sexual lives. Therefore, the same sex-related parts that can cause the host so much trouble during adulthood may have helped provide her with a fighting chance to finally enter a healthy sexual relationship with all of her mind.

POINTS TO KEEP IN MIND

- Sexually aggressive parts act according to trauma-related needs and do not intend to cause harm.

- Knowing why sexual parts are active helps the host and her loved ones understand and empathize with all her parts.

- All parts can gradually learn that sex can be a choice and a nonabusive pleasure.

8

SEXUAL PARTNERSHIPS

[Knowing that a partner has parts] puts a huge burden on the other person that I can't even begin to understand.

—Gabbi

◉

In a long-term partnership, a diagnosis of DID can fall like a wedge, splitting the relationship into "before diagnosis" and "after diagnosis." The difference between before and after is simply the difference between knowing and not knowing that the person has parts. Yet, what a difference knowing can make. My interviewees show that years of living together can pass during which neither the woman nor her partner is aware that a woman has parts: she thinks that her experiences are the norm or just the way she is; her partner may know and then be puzzled by her behavior but otherwise notices nothing. This holds true whether parts are sexually active or not, and whether a woman's partner is male or female. The other parts who are active in the outside world can generally pass as the host, and the host's partner, like most people, is likely to assume unity in a person's memory and perceptions and therefore find them.

If traumatic memories and noticeably different parts begin emerging, the experience can frighten both partners and shake the partnership.[1] Some research has mentioned disruptions of sexual partnerships caused by parts,[2] and among my interviewees, parts' disruptive behavior has affected the partnerships of four out of the six women who are or have been in long-term sexual partnerships. A part can pick fights, attack a partner, and have sex outside the partnership, causing quarrels, jealousy, fear, battery, and divorce.

Some parts may deny having a partner at all and see no reason to behave nicely to the person with whom she or he lives. A part may consistently displease a partner because her or his character differs widely from the host's. It is striking that in all these disruptions, neither partner may recognize or even suspect the actual cause of such behavior.

BEFORE THE DIAGNOSIS: "WE NEVER TALKED ABOUT IT"

Ellie's marriage is an example of mutual oblivion. Her husband, Joe, was simply puzzled by the way Ellie would sometimes sit on the floor and play with toys, an activity she, as the host, could not remember. Ellie and Joe were both baffled by her occasional ambivalence about having sex, simultaneously wanting to and not wanting to. Puzzling, too, was her fear of driving down certain roads while on vacation, a fear only later recognized as stemming from memories of places where childhood abuse had occurred.

Similarly, Samantha's second husband, John, noticed that she would sometimes act "really weird," as Samantha put it, "like, get all scared for no reason and run away for no reason, and try to kill myself for no reason. . . . He thought I was acting crazy." Even while noticing her obviously distressing behavior, John was unaware that he was speaking with separated parts of his wife's mind on a regular basis, especially with a part called The Smart One. Samantha met John as a fellow lawyer at work; therefore, he first knew her as The Smart One, the intellectual part of Samantha's mind. Even at home, John knew mainly The Smart One because so much had to be done quickly and only The Smart One could accomplish household tasks quickly enough. "So she would just take over almost everybody's jobs; and she would be the one talking," Samantha said. Other parts would then be switched into control of the body, depending on what type of talk would best suit John's immediate needs. Samantha described such a switch:

My ex-husband and I were discussing something, and he was talking to
The Smart One. She was making him really mad 'cause she was being
businesslike about it, [and] he didn't want it to be businesslike. So we
switched Julia out so that she could be nice. She got him to calm down
so he wasn't mad anymore.

Unbeknownst to him, John never had sex with the parts of his wife's
mind he usually talked with, but with the fourteen-year-old part called
Cecelia. John, occasionally perplexed by Samantha's "really weird" behavior, was oblivious to the extremely subtle but daily changes of identity that
happened before his eyes.

Samantha's first husband may have known more. Cecelia, the part who
takes care of sex, told me that he found out that "there were other people
there, and he was glad 'cause he could get people to come out [and] do bad
things." When I asked Cecelia if she would give an example of the "bad
things," she declined, and when I asked her if he understood that he was
eliciting other parts, she said she did not know: "We never talked about it."
They could not have discussed it because, at the time, Samantha did not
know that there were other parts; she only knew that she heard voices and
assumed that was the norm. Samantha's first husband belonged to what
Samantha called a "satanic cult," to which he reportedly took Samantha
and where he may have seen how she could be manipulated. Possibly he
knew about dissociated parts; certainly he knew that he could make his wife
do his bidding, however distorted his requests might be.

Neither of Elizabeth's husbands was aware that only part of the Elizabeth they knew was governing her body during sex. Yet her first husband,
who was physically and emotionally abusive, took advantage of Elizabeth's
dissociated state without realizing it. He did whatever he wished with her
body and was pleased to have a wife so acquiescent. Indeed, sexual parts
affected Elizabeth's and Samantha's first marriages in ways that well-suited
their abusive partners and perhaps strengthened the marital bonds,
unhealthy as they were.

During Elizabeth's and Samantha's marriages, their sexual parts never actively sought out other men. Perhaps they felt the commitment to monogamy and/or felt sufficiently active and useful within the marriage. In contrast, Caroline's sexual part, Terry, was not monogamous whether Caroline was married or single. Terry may have never considered herself married. Parts who consider a spouse "*her* husband, not mine" are frequently the cause of sexual infidelity among women who have sexually active parts.[3] Also, Terry needed to repeatedly reverse her childhood trauma by feeling in control of men, as Caroline explained. Caroline's first husband never noticed, being away most of the time. Bob, her second husband, eventually found out about Caroline's sexual unfaithfulness, a discovery that shook the marriage for years and created lasting tension.

> It embarrasses me. . . . We had a personality that was very promiscuous, and we had affairs with a lot of different people. . . . [Bob] found out at some point in my life about an affair that I had with someone. After that, he would accuse us constantly of having affairs with this one, that one. It wasn't even true; we'd had one with someone but certainly not with everybody that he was thinking. That was a hard time for a lot of us.

Caroline thinks that Terry "went into hiding" after that affair, but her language reveals an uncertainty about those memories. "I think that it was all accusations from my husband with no basis after that. I don't know; that's still all foggy." Even now that Caroline knows Terry is no longer sexually active, Bob's suspicion lingers, and Caroline's statements concerning her whereabouts are greeted with disbelief. "If I tell him that I went to the mall, he'll just stare at me, trying to say, 'You really didn't go there. I know you were probably somewhere else,' when I *was* at the mall. It's really annoying."

As three of my interviewees have learned, sexual parts' various desires and needs can shake or destroy a relationship with neither partner understanding the true cause. When inner communication and cooperation have not yet been achieved, it is impossible for the host to negotiate with other parts of the mind to try to find a compromise, to make internal decisions beneficial to the partnership, or to have all parts agree to be in a relationship. Before diagnosis, the host is not likely to realize that one or more other parts of her mind are causing the destructive behavior. Diagnosis and skilled therapy can improve such a situation. Yet, even though therapy can facilitate greater inner cooperation, the diagnosis itself can burden the relationship.

After Diagnosis

One can appreciate a person's shock on learning after years of living together that most parts of a partner's mind are not conscious during sex. Even the most understanding and composed partner must blanch at the knowledge that a beloved person has identities who are children or who are adult males who refuse to acknowledge the bond. Indeed, my interviewees illustrate the power of the diagnosis over the partnership. No other diagnosis of psychological distress is so likely to change both partners' perceptions of the diagnosed person.

With an accurate diagnosis comes therapy, during which traumatic childhood experiences may be put into words and shared with other parts, causing unwillingness to have sex, or more activity among the parts that held traumatic memories. Scenes on the nuptial bed can become nightmarish if a terrified child part takes over a woman's body and perceives all lovemaking as assault or rape.

Amidst the emotional turmoil, a partner's reaction to a diagnosis is crucial because it can affect both the partnership and the outcome of therapy. Ideally, a partner's attitude and behavior would include the following:

- A concern for the diagnosed person that encompasses all parts of her mind (as opposed to excluding one or more parts or becoming fascinated by them)

- Immediate acceptance of all signs of sexual unwillingness; no insistent sexual approaches

- Moderate, not intrusive, curiosity about a woman's past or about the material discussed in therapy[4]

Such acceptance, combined with moderation, is much to ask of even the most devoted partner. My interviewees' partners are no exceptions.

Caroline and Bob: "I Wish He Never Knew"

Caroline's husband, Bob, is one example. Bob was ambivalent about learning of his wife's diagnosis, or perhaps simply not interested. Caroline first tried to lead up to the subject, leaving books on dissociative disorders lying around the house, hoping he would ask why she was so interested in the subject. To no avail.

> I had to really tell him. But he's one of these people that you tell something and he'll say, "Oh, yeah, okay. What are we having for supper?" But then he'll say, "Well, you never told me." And I'll say, "I tried to tell you; you don't want to listen." "That's not true, I want to listen." So I say, "Okay, I'll tell you." So I'll start to tell him again, and he'll say, "Well, I have to be in to work at six in the morning." He just doesn't want to know about it.

In spite of Bob's reluctance to know, Caroline's information did make an impression on him. Since learning of the diagnosis, Bob sometimes stares at her as though waiting for her to switch. "I hate that," Caroline says, "I wish he never knew." When Caroline is angry with him, he now blames the anger on another part of her mind, frustrating Caroline by denying her strong feelings. "We are *all* mad; you're a jerk," she says, re-creating the moment and emphasizing that her whole being is angry. Bob is also sometimes sarcastic, telling her how silly he thinks she looks when youthful parts influence her wholehearted play with their grandchildren. "I just blast him a look," Caroline says, implying that her killing glance is enough to silence him, at least for the time being. Caroline's description suggests that Bob's reactions fall well short of optimal on at least three counts: he has little concern about or interest in Caroline's welfare related to DID; he ridicules her child parts when they influence play; and he shows no curiosity about Caroline's past or about her experiences in therapy. However, he appears to understand the diagnosis well enough to use DID as a way of denying that Caroline's negative feelings toward him are her own.

Ellie and Joe: "She Hasn't Wanted Me to Be Married"

Ellie's husband, Joe, was initially skeptical about the diagnosis, interpreting it as Ellie's "convenient" way of excusing all inappropriate or disagreeable behavior, past, present, and future. Joe then met with Ellie's therapist, and he left the session believing the diagnosis. Knowing the diagnosis has affected their relationship more than Ellie's parts ever did. The effects have been mainly positive. For example, the diagnosis helped Joe understand Ellie's occasional sexual reticence. Her initial stiffness and sense of "I don't want to do this" usually goes away during sex, but if it does not, she tells Joe, "This is not a good time," and most often he understands.

The reason behind Ellie's occasional reluctance is Myra, the lesbian part of Ellie's mind. Myra is an example of a part who disavows a marriage. Sometimes, such a part will even leave home when in control of the body.[5] Although Myra has never left home, she has sometimes been difficult for Ellie to cope with.

> She hasn't wanted me to be married; she hasn't wanted me to be in relationships with men. She has wanted to be the one in control of our sex life. [Ellie laughingly gives an example of her quarrels with Myra:]

"Sorry, I've chosen *this* partner; *this* is the way it's going to be!" So that has been a difficult part for my husband and for me to deal with. He's not real fond of *her* either.

In spite of their mutual dislike, Joe says that he does not much mind Myra as long as she stays quietly inside.

Joe has also learned to be tolerant of Ellie's occasional childlike behavior, as long as it occurs within the privacy of home. If Ellie's child part, Jesse, wants to play alone or with Ellie's granddaughter, Joe understands that it is best to let Jesse play. Joe shows his care for Ellie partly by protecting her from inappropriate behavior in public, quietly insisting that she leave any toylike figures alone. Speaking of a party in a relative's home, Ellie explained, "It wasn't that I didn't realize that it was inappropriate behavior; I *did*. It's just [that] there was such a strong need to play with those things." If he has seen Ellie playing with toys for a while at home, Joe is less apt to be romantic. Joe's reticence at such times is wise. "He feels it's like having sex with a child when I'm in that mode," Ellie said.

Now that Ellie's traumatic memories have been worked through with her therapist and other parts are generally quiescent and cooperative, Ellie and Joe can see the humor in some of their unique situations as a couple. Joe knows there is significance in how Ellie takes her morning coffee: black or with cream and sugar. "He goes, 'Okay, what's it going to be today?' [and I'll say,] 'I'm going to have it black today.' He goes [Ellie barely holds back her laughter], 'Okay, I just wanted to know who I was dealing with.'" Her toys are another source of laughter, and Ellie has a collection that fills the house. Now and then she tries using her granddaughter as an excuse to buy more toys, a ploy Joe immediately sees through. Even Ellie's lesbian part Myra is a source of a standing joke between husband and wife.

She came out one time at the mall. I'll never forget it because I couldn't control what she was saying. She was walking, well, *I* was walking with Joe through the mall, and a particularly good-looking girl walked by. Joe turned to look at the girl and I, Myra, or whoever, grabbed him by the arm and spun him around. He thought that I was going to say, "Quit looking at other women!" And what actually came out of my mouth was, "Hey, I saw her first!" And he was like, "What!" He was *not* pleased to hear me saying something like that in public. Almost as soon as he said "what," Myra retreated, and there I was to face his questions. It was actually kind of funny. He brings that up every now and then, and he'll say to me, "Hey, I saw her first!" [Ellie and I laugh.]

Joe shows himself an optimal partner: he is not insistent on sex if Ellie is unwilling, protects Ellie in public, and even (reluctantly) accepts Myra rather than rejects her or any other parts of Ellie's mind. Joe shows concern for and acceptance of Ellie as a whole person, including her lesbian tendencies and her occasional childlike playfulness. He accepts her childlike actions as long as they do not publicly endanger her image as a singleton. Joe also illustrates that a sense of humor about having parts can disperse possible tensions. Sharing jokes about Ellie's occasionally unusual behavior seems to help bind the couple together. Whenever an attractive woman passes and Joe says to Ellie, "Hey, I saw her first," they are sharing a joke they created. The two of them understand the suffering and struggle behind that joke.

Gabbi and Sue: "I Have to Give Her a Whole Lot of Credit"

Gabbi lives with her lesbian partner of twenty-one years. Before her diagnosis, Gabbi and her partner, Sue, had standing jokes about Gabbi's memory lapses and uncharacteristic behavior. However, their humor simply hid the uneasiness and fear both of them felt about the possible meaning of Gabbi's behavior. "Scary" seems to be a key word for Gabbi, one she often repeated in conjunction with DID. Having dissociated identities is scary, as was disclosing her diagnosis to her partner. Gabbi feared that disclosure would change the relationship, a fear she shares with other women in similar situations.[6]

You know, there is some risk that it's going to affect things, that it's not going to be accepted, not going to be understood. That's a therapist's job. If there was anybody in the world that was going to be okay to tell, that would be the person. They're trained in that, and they see all kinds of abnormal things. Your partner doesn't. They're not used to seeing that kind of stuff.

Gabbi thinks that Sue did not want to know the truth anyway. Having an abuse background of her own, Sue does not like talking about emotions or the past so that Gabbi's struggles are uncomfortably "close to home" for Sue. Also, like most people, Sue is not used to hearing about "abnormal" conditions. Gabbi also admits that she herself was afraid to know much about her own states of mind. Consequently, although Gabbi learned of her diagnosis four years after she met Sue, she waited another thirteen years before telling her. For seventeen years both Gabbi and Sue accommodated Gabbi's occasionally strange behavior by brushing it off and treating it humorously. Gabbi eventually disclosed to Sue during a time when Gabbi was having much difficulty functioning. The disclosure was part of Gabbi's own questions about herself: "How do [I] get better? Where do [I] go from here? What's the future? Is it fixable or have I lost my mind and am going to be institutionalized for the rest of my life?"

Knowing the diagnosis enables Gabbi and Sue to discuss the condition, and Sue can now make allowances for some of Gabbi's behavior, seeking help when necessary. Sue recognizes a switch by marked changes in Gabbi's speech and behavior, and now knows other parts of Gabbi's mind. Sue used to argue or fight with some of them, making the situation worse. Now she recognizes when other parts are in control and does not bother to quarrel with them. "She just lets it go, 'cause she knows it isn't me," Gabbi says. About every other day, Sue has to talk to younger parts of Gabbi's mind rather than to Gabbi, the adult host, and sometimes finds herself with a younger part during sex. Sue then immediately ceases the sexual intimacy. "She's totally uncomfortable with it," Gabbi said. "As soon as she knows that's happening, it's basically over. She's not interested in having that level of a relationship with anybody else." There are times when Sue gets very tired of it all and, understandably, wants Gabbi to simply be the adult Gabbi she knows best. However, the diagnosis helped Gabbi and Sue understand Gabbi's ambivalence about preferring women or men, just as the diagnosis helped Ellie and her husband, Joe. Sexual ambivalence is a trait Gabbi and Ellie share with countless women and men who have dissociated identities.[7]

Sue does not know much about Gabbi's ongoing one-night stands with men when a part of Gabbi's mind goes out in search of abusive sex. Sue does, however, know that she is Gabbi's sole lesbian relationship and that Gabbi has only recently wanted to think of herself as having any sort of sexual preference or interest, with that interest being increasingly heterosexual. Such changes in sexual identity can occur when parts of a person's mind begin to unify. Sometimes such a change terminates a long-term relationship if its sexual orientation is no longer the person's own.[8] Gabbi's change and ambiguity are clear to Sue and she tolerates them, not asking for more information and getting little because Gabbi does not want to needlessly hurt her.

Caregiving is also now a part of Sue's life. Her love and her knowledge of the diagnosis have led her to spend much time monitoring Gabbi. Like a mother with one eye always on her child, Sue keeps track of Gabbi's whereabouts and watches how she speaks and behaves. She plans ahead for likely switches by being aware of stressful situations in Gabbi's life, knowing that Gabbi is more easily triggered when she cannot sleep, when she has a difficult time in therapy, and when her work is stressful and unusually long. When Gabbi has switched, Sue talks with Gabbi's therapist and together they try to get Gabbi to therapy quickly so that she, as her adult, professional self, can regain control of her body and save her job as a director of finance and administration specializing in health care.

When Gabbi has to go to a work-related party, she is relieved when Sue is present. Yet, Sue cannot completely relax at the party or concentrate on other people. She is constantly vigilant, watching Gabbi and ready to take her back to the safety of home at a moment's notice.

We've been together twenty-one years . . . so she knows me well enough
to know who I am and what my habits are. She just pays attention to
my interactions with people, how comfortable I am. Am I talking? Am
I not talking? Am I withdrawing to the corner of the room? Am I hiding in the ladies' room? If I'm out and looking comfortable and talking
to people, then I'm okay. She watches how much I drink. Do I start
drinking? ['cause I don't drink;] do I start smoking? 'cause I don't smoke;
do I start dancing with men? 'cause I don't dance with men—but there
are personalities that do.

Gabbi is aware of Sue's strength and sacrifices and is grateful for them.
After posing many specific questions, I asked Gabbi to tell me what else
concerning relationships might come to her mind. She immediately began
a verbal tribute to her partner:

I think relationships are difficult by nature. You've got two people with
different interests and values trying to come together. And we further
complicate that by having six people that have to compromise, get
along, and share. It puts a huge burden on the other person that I can't
even begin to understand because I'm not in that other position. From
my point of view, I know how hard a one-on-one relationship is. We've
worked hard to understand each other and make our relationship good
and make it work and be strong. I have to give her a whole lot of credit
'cause I think she's had a much tougher job than I've had. Just being
flexible enough to adjust to what she needed to and not take on too
much that had nothing to do with our [relationship]. And maybe that's
one of the things she is so good at: staying out of and not thinking a
whole lot about human behavior and what's happening. She probably
would have gone crazy if she spent a lot of time doing that as opposed
to, "We're just going to go to the movies. And if I go to the movies with
you or if I go with somebody else, we're going to go to the movies and
we're going to have fun." You know what I mean?

Gabbi considers herself fortunate to have found someone who is capable of taking on the complexities and challenges of living with a person who has unruly parts. Gabbi marvels that all of her friends are separated or divorced, yet she and Sue, with their abusive backgrounds and turbulent daily lives, have held together for over two decades. "I look around and other than [my sister], I don't know anybody that's still together, or people that don't struggle with these kinds of things under the best of circumstances." Indeed, people who have no dissociated parts but are struggling to keep their partnerships together can see some of their own problems as similar but multiplied by having parts. Two people, but several identities, each with distinct character traits and preferences, have to "compromise, get along, and share."

Although Sue's reactions may be partly based on fear or denial, she exemplifies the behavior shown to be crucial for a partnership: concern for Gabbi and for all parts of her mind, and restraint in both sexuality and curiosity about Gabbi's condition and about her past. Gabbi knows the value of this approach and applauds Sue for trying to live without concern as much as possible rather than getting needlessly involved and troubled, realizing that at times, it may be better not to analyze human behavior.

Elizabeth and David: "I Left Them So They Could Have a Better Life"

Elizabeth divorced her abusive first husband and remarried, still without knowing about the dissociated parts of her mind. During her second marriage, Elizabeth was once hospitalized for depression, suicidal wishes, and self-injury, during which time she was diagnosed as having DID. After her return home, she told her husband, David, that she had what was then called multiple personalities, and hospital staff explained to David the meaning of Elizabeth's diagnosis. David reacted calmly and seemed understanding, saying that the diagnosis made sense of some behavior that used to confuse him. "He said, 'Yeah, I can see that.' 'Cause he said sometimes I was really nasty, and other times there was no sign of that."

The blow fell later, when the couple decided to divorce, with the understanding that Elizabeth and their two children would stay in the condominium where they lived and David would move out, visit the children on a regular basis, and pay child support. One day, shortly after this decision, Elizabeth tried to pay the paper boy, only to discover that there was no money in the bank. When she asked David about it, he said, "Oh yeah, I closed out all the accounts two weeks ago, they're all in my name. You don't have a penny, and you need to leave." Then came the pronouncement that changed Elizabeth's life.

> The threat was that I wouldn't have any contact with the kids. He said that he [would] tell in court how I'm an unfit mother because I have multiple personalities and I would never see my kids. And [he said] that my father, this man in a pretty high position in state government, would be exposed for the history of my childhood. Both of those threats were very serious to me. And so I agreed for him to have physical custody so I could have visitations and see my children. The other choice was that I would never see my kids again. So, I had not a penny, no place to live, he would drag it through court and drag the kids through court—and I could not and would not put my children on the stand at court. So I—[pause because she cries] left them so they could have a better life.

In order to prevent her childhood abuse and diagnosis, so private and painful, from being exposed in public with her children as witnesses, and in order to at least be granted parental visitation rights, Elizabeth gave up physical custody of her children. Simply the knowledge of her diagnosis gave her husband this power over her life and over their children's lives. Even though the actual parenting ability of the mother, not her diagnosis, should determine whether she has custody, some women refuse to let a partner be informed of a diagnosis, fearing that the information might be used against them.[9] Elizabeth had to experience the reality behind those women's fears. The forced renunciation of her children's daily presence left Elizabeth in a state of suicidal anguish for years.

Samantha and John: "With John We Could Be Who We Were"

Like Elizabeth, Samantha divorced her abusive first husband and remarried, all without knowing about the other parts of her mind. After years of marriage to her second husband, John, Samantha was finally correctly diagnosed, and her therapist explained the diagnosis to John. For a while, John went with Samantha to her therapy sessions, becoming very involved in her therapy and learning about all parts of her mind. His reaction to what he learned was mainly heightened interest. "He was more curious than anything about what it meant and who all was there. . . . He made a point of finding out when somebody new had come out, getting to know everybody [by] talking to them and asking them about themselves." This process interested Samantha because she listened to what the other parts told John and learned, with him, about their functions and characteristics.

> There's one who's four and she likes ice cream. So he would buy her ice cream every now and then and play with her. He bought some blocks [and] they'd play with blocks while she ate her ice cream.

Yet, John's curiosity also made Samantha uncomfortable: "I felt like if I'm supposed to be just one person, then he should be treating me like I'm one person instead of making a big deal out of each part." Samantha instinctively knew the dangers of becoming fascinated by parts rather than concerned for the diagnosed person as a whole.

Indeed, John's knowledge of her diagnosis weakened the marriage by making Samantha a sideshow for him instead of the person who before was simply his wife. "It messed everything up with John. It turned into what we talked about most of the time, and he was always trying to figure out what was going on instead of just living." Rather than concern for Samantha as the sum of all her parts, John seems to have become intrigued by the phenomenon of dissociated parts and lost sight of the Samantha he had known.

John's knowledge of the diagnosis also changed the couple's sexual life, at least temporarily. John was unhappy that his sexual relationship was only with one part of Samantha, not with her as a whole person. Moreover, he learned that the part of Samantha's mind with whom he was making love is fourteen, and he thought that too young for sex. John seems to have been embarrassed that others should know that he was sleeping with an adolescent whose main function is having sex. That adolescent's name used to be The One Who Performs Sexual Functions. John made her change her name "'cause he said he didn't want her telling anybody that was her name," Samantha said. When I spoke with Cecelia, as the sexual part is now called, she said that sex was "weird" for a while after John learned about her. "At first he was real standoffish, and then he wanted sex more than usual." Finding out about Cecelia changed John's attitude and behavior toward the same sexual relationship he had always known.

John's reactions evidently subsided over time, and he eventually came to terms with the new knowledge about his wife. Then later, during a volatile time, a malevolent male part who hated John attacked him with a knife, then tried to strangle him, incidents that shook both partners. Also, because of repeated suicide attempts, Samantha entered a two-month hospital program. During that time, John was upset about her absence and turned his interest to another woman. "Then he just left," Samantha said. "I was very hurt, 'cause we'd gone through so much together that it's hard to believe that he'd leave." John explained his leaving as the result of the crises and changes caused by DID. "He said he just couldn't stand it anymore." Samantha felt that the most important negative effect of DID on her life was its role in the dissolution of her second marriage.

> With John we could be who we were. We didn't have to be careful whose
> voice was coming out or whether somebody was saying something age-

inappropriate, because he knew all of us and he could deal with it. John is the only one who knows Samantha, [and] he knew me and loved me when he thought I was just Samantha. And then he left me alone with all these people.

Samantha's view of her husband's departure has a unique poignancy. Only John knew and loved her both before and after her diagnosis. She and John had learned together that Samantha alone is different from Samantha as the sum of her parts, making him the only person in her private life who truly "knows Samantha." Only with him could she be her whole self and be accepted, making his loss feel irreparable. Also, coming so soon after her diagnosis, the divorce left her feeling abandoned with her new sense of herself as only one part alone with all her "people."

THE IMPACT OF A DIAGNOSIS

According to my interviewees, none of their partners suspected that they had been living with someone who has parts,[10] and the diagnosis changed every long-term relationship. Ironically, it is the perceived identity of both partners that is changed by such important new information. Discovery that a partner is having an affair can mean "You are not the faithful, trustworthy person who loves only me, as I believed you were; and I am not the sole beloved and partner of your life, as I believed I was." This sudden, dual loss of identity is a major part of the devastation an extramarital affair can cause. Discovering that one's partner has a mind in dissociated parts can have a similar effect, changing the perceived identity of the diagnosed partner forever. Only this time the change is not always from one identity to another but from one identity to an open question: "Who are you?" asks the partner, and "Who am I?" asks the diagnosed person.

Nonetheless, this profound change can be for the better even if improvement in mutual understanding comes only after a long struggle. Through knowing about parts and their origins, both partners can understand previously puzzling behaviors such as sexual ambivalence, forgetfulness, childlike play, or suicide attempts. Armed with their new knowledge, partners can discuss their problems and realize that their situation requires a high level of understanding and tolerance. Ellie's and Gabbi's partners rose to the challenge. Ellie's husband, Joe, seems to have been mainly understanding and tolerant, taking Ellie's love of toys and attractive women with a healthy sense of humor. Gabbi's partner, Sue, cares for Gabbi during her frequent switches, conveying information to Gabbi's therapist and planning ahead for stressful times. Sue and Joe choose to go without sex rather than make love to obviously inappropriate parts of their partners' minds. Both of them quietly protect their partners from public notice and embarrassment.

However, when partners become estranged, the question, "Who are you?" can become, "How can I take advantage of her diagnosis to my benefit?" Therefore, women who have dissociated identities are caught between two disquieting possibilities. They can either endure the emotional isolation of keeping the diagnosis a secret from their partners or risk having the diagnosis used against them. Elizabeth, Samantha, and Caroline opened doors to their inner worlds and let their partners peek in. Because of their partners' reactions to what they saw, all three women regret that they told their husbands about the many parts of their minds.

Having a Second Chance

When new information damages a partnership irreparably, the lessons learned can be put to good use with a new partner. Three of the women I interviewed have had such a chance. Samantha's opportunity came after her second divorce, when Samantha was hoping to find a man with whom she could have a lasting relationship. I asked her a hypothetical question: If she became serious about someone, would she tell that person about her diagnosis? Her reply was, "I don't think I would tell him ever." Her response did not surprise me because I knew that she blamed the dissolution of her second marriage on the knowledge of her diagnosis and on disruptions caused by having parts. Ten months after the original interview, I talked with Samantha again to clarify some points. I found that she had indeed become serious about someone else, someone she had met via the Internet. The Internet meeting took place with serendipitous timing. Samantha was sitting at her computer, about to delete her ad for a serious partner because the ad was still attracting men interested only in sex.

> Just then a message came in saying, "I'd like to know if you have [twelve] kids, when you had time for law school." And I thought, "Well, that doesn't sound like somebody just for sex." So we answered the ad and that was Bill—and then we deleted the ad.

Before her marriage to Bill, Samantha struggled with the question of disclosing her diagnosis, fearing that disclosure would destroy her chance of building a healthy, durable partnership.

> I didn't want to tell him 'cause I thought he wouldn't marry me if I told him. Then I prayed about it, and I decided that it was wrong to marry somebody without telling them something as essential as that. So we told him. He asked if [it meant] he was going to be polygamous. [Samantha and I laugh heartily.]

Samantha decided that a lifelong commitment should not begin with secrecy, and that knowing her diagnosis obliged her to disclose it to a prospective husband. Bill did not change his mind, and the two married. Bill has asked Samantha to tell him more "about everybody" or to write about them when she feels comfortable doing so. This request pleases Samantha because she perceives it as showing that Bill is not inclined to make Samantha's partitioned mind a focus, but is simply interested in knowing more about his wife. Also, Bill's humor, like the humor of Ellie's husband, Joe, may help both Bill and Samantha in future years.

Elizabeth is equally pleased with her new partnership. After divorces from two husbands, Elizabeth gradually found herself falling in love with a woman, Peggy, with whom she now lives. Early in their acquaintanceship, Elizabeth told Peggy about her parts. Peggy had been through depression and therapy and had known something about dissociative identity disorder. After Elizabeth spoke with her, Peggy researched the topic and developed a better understanding of it. Elizabeth characterizes Peggy's response as "very supportive all around."

> [She said] that it was okay, that she understood. And later on, when we decided to have a more permanent relationship and live together, we agreed to seek out therapy or couples counseling if there was any difficulty in our relationship. So we had [my] therapy, her therapy, and our therapy as needed, [and] everybody knew [about] DID.

Elizabeth and Peggy decided to be always willing to talk about DID, as they still do whenever necessary. Peggy would see major changes in Elizabeth and tell Elizabeth what she saw. Some parts of Elizabeth's mind were more pleasant to meet than others, but Peggy was patient with the unpleasant ones and indulgent to the others, and meeting them helped her understand them. When contentious parts became mean and instigated fights, Peggy would try to talk to the Elizabeth she knew best or to the contentious part and manage the situation herself. Alternatively, Peggy would simply remove herself from the situation, telling the unruly part to call the therapist: "Time to call Sonja. I'm going out now, are you all right in the house? Don't leave the house; call Sonja." The most difficult times for Peggy were finding that Elizabeth had cut or burned herself again. Peggy would not tolerate Elizabeth's self-injury, and the problem brought the two of them to counseling together. Such trying times no longer occur now that Elizabeth's feelings no longer overwhelm her.

When Elizabeth's child parts wanted to be playful, Peggy entertained them, sitting on the floor playing jacks, or playing with dolls or cutouts. Peggy would monitor Elizabeth so that she could go to a toy store, an amusement park, or the zoo and let child parts emerge. "I could actually *be* that child and start to feel it myself," Elizabeth says. Elizabeth now considers herself healthier because she was able to allow her other parts more time in control, thanks to Peggy's positive attitude. At toy stores, Peggy would say either, "Yes, you can get that doll," or "No, not today." The child parts were always excited and bubbly, having never been allowed to play before, so the couple spent a few years playing "a lot." The experience of being a safe, playful child allowed some of the child parts to grow up and mature. After a while, the need to be a child dwindled and now emerges only occasionally.

> Once in a while, we'll say, "Oh, let's go be kids, fool around, ride our bikes somewhere or ride our scooters"—two forty-three-year-olds on their scooters, with helmets—all right, not the most enjoyable sight. But we'll go to a park and do that and not care what anyone thinks, just be goofy and have fun.

Like Elizabeth, Lucy also has found an understanding and knowledgeable new partner, a fellow therapist named Jennifer. The two women had known each other as friends, and Lucy had told Jennifer about the diagnosis. Jennifer's response was, "Oh, that makes sense," commenting that she finally understood why sometimes Lucy would forget to meet with her. When they became seriously interested in each other as partners, Lucy insisted that Jennifer see Lucy's therapist to learn everything she could about Lucy's inner situation and her behavior. Lucy had suffered when a previous partner left because of Lucy's parts. Lucy learned caution from that experience. "It's like, 'Look, if we're going to do this, you need to know this now.'" Only when Jennifer had gone over every aspect of Lucy's condition with the therapist and accepted them was Lucy willing to talk with Jennifer about the possibility of living together.

Lucy is now rewarded with a partner who seems to enjoy all parts of Lucy's mind, including the irrepressible Rose, a child part of indeterminate age who conducted roughly half of the interview with me. I could tell when

Rose was speaking during the long-distance interview because of her child-like, playful vocal tone and pitch and her unique grammar. Because of Rose and other energetic parts, Jennifer never has a dull moment. Lucy constantly has new ideas, youthful questions, and new ways of seeing things. Lucy also has a knack for doing at least two things simultaneously: brushing her teeth and drying her hair; dusting, sweeping, and talking on the telephone. Lucy has to be reminded that Jennifer can only do one thing at a time, and Lucy takes pity on Jennifer's disadvantage: "She's a singleton."

All three women who met their partners after diagnosis experienced the same circumstances favorable to a relationship. They had had at least a few years of therapy so that they understood their behavior and had been able to modify it to some degree for smoother functioning. Also, the three women and their partners were forewarned and therefore came together prepared to face DID as part of their tasks in partnership. Two of the women's partners have utilized therapeutic help or organized it for possible future needs. This preparation depended on the women with parts risking rejection by disclosing the diagnosis to their prospective partners at the outset. The opportunity to work together with their partners on the unique challenges that lay ahead made the risk worth taking. Finally, their partners immediately accepted the diagnosis as valid, and their ongoing responses largely correspond to the three crucial aspects of a supportive reaction outlined earlier:

1. They relate to all the identities to whom they are introduced without rejecting, exploiting, or becoming fascinated by them or making them a focus.
2. Their sexual approaches are not frightening or insistent.
3. Their curiosity about the partner's past or about the material she discusses in therapy is moderate.[11]

My interviewees' and their partners' experiences further support the importance of these guidelines when the existence of dissociated parts is revealed. These guidelines, along with an unflagging mutual commitment and good-natured humor, can help a couple survive the tremor of a DID diagnosis midway in a partnership, and they can strengthen the bond of those who knew at the beginning.

POINTS TO KEEP IN MIND

- The guidelines outlined in this chapter can help a person learn how to react in helpful ways to the knowledge of a partner's dissociated parts.

- For a person who has parts, there are benefits and risks involved in disclosing the diagnosis to a partner, but the risks may not reveal themselves for years.

- The changed perception of a person's identity that accompanies a diagnosis can cause as much or more upheaval than the parts themselves.

- Partners of people who have DID may be helped through support groups or therapists well-versed in dissociative disorders to understand the meaning of having dissociated identities and discuss questions about trust, sex, parenting, caring for oneself, appropriate responses to various parts, and problems that arise in everyday life.

- Unknown numbers of couples go through life without either partner recognizing the presence of dissociated parts.

9

PARENTING WITH PARTS

I regret to this day that I hadn't gone through therapy before having children. What was I thinking!
—*Ellie, a forty-three-year-old retail manager*

⊙

Ellie's statement reveals a mother's lifelong remorse at the suffering she may have inadvertently caused during her children's crucial years of development. Such concern can plague a parent diagnosed with DID, some of whom have mentioned a child's fright at a sudden, noticeable change in voice, speech, or looks[1] and ruefully recounted a child's endurance of uncontrollable beatings, yelling, emotional neglect, inconsistent behavior, and age-inappropriate demands on the child.[2] Dissociation has been linked to parents' problems with showing affection or with using supportive discipline.[3] In addition, a parent's suicide attempts and hospitalizations cause painful separations and a child's fear of permanent loss. Cases of child abuse by a parent or stepparent who has parts are known among therapists who specialize in DID.[4]

Uneasiness on the child's behalf may be the first reaction when other people hear that a parent has DID. Indeed, motherhood is perhaps the most emotionally laden topic related to women who have parts. How are all parts treating the children? Do the children notice anything unusual about their mother's behavior? Do the children know about the diagnosis, and if they know, how are they coping with this knowledge? What helps a mother who has DID be a good parent? These questions are particularly pressing for two reasons. First, the majority of people in therapy for DID are women in their childbearing and child-rearing years.[5] Second, dissociation may be a factor that determines why some formerly abused parents abuse their own children and others do not.[6] Dissociation of all types seems to be a link between a mother's own childhood abuse and her risk of inconsistent discipline, physical neglect, and use of physical punishment on her children.[7]

Some women who are struggling with having dissociated parts and other effects of childhood abuse decide to remain childless temporarily or permanently, fearing that their children might suffer. Because countless women, however, are never correctly diagnosed, or remain undiagnosed well into adulthood, they bear and raise children long before they become acquainted with the term *dissociative identity disorder*. This was the case with the four parents I interviewed, Caroline, Samantha, Ellie, and Elizabeth, and for the stepparent Lucy. Only Reba had begun therapy for DID before the niece and nephew under her care were born.

These six women are trying to escape their own parents' model of parenthood. They want other parts of their minds to help them function so that they can be good caregivers. They are trying to suppress aspects of DID inimical to good parenting. Those aspects include the following:

- Parts who do not consider themselves mothers and are neglectful, irresponsible, persecutory, or rageful

- Parts who act as parents but whose standards are vastly different from the host's standards

- Short- or long-term memory loss of parenting experiences

- Parts who self-injure, are depressed, or attempt suicide

In the following section, these women discuss the obstacles DID can place in a parent's way. They introduce the parts who have talents as parents and those who do not, and show when the instinct to protect and nurture their children prevails and when and why it fails.

MISSING MEMORIES OF MOTHERHOOD

Anything to do with kids, I'm lost.

—Caroline

Fifty-seven-year-old Caroline and I faced a dilemma: I began asking about her experiences as a mother only to find that her memory of her children's younger years is currently irretrievable. She explained to me that most of the time, a combination of two female parts called Pam and Jessica was talking to me during the interview. During Caroline's teenage years, a part called Terry was active along with Pam and Jessica. The Terry part of Caroline's mind controlled her sexual life and slept with several men. Caroline became pregnant at fifteen and married. When she gave birth at sixteen, the Pam and Jessica parts "faded out," and a complete or partial memory blackout began for those parts that lasted until Caroline was thirty-six. Caroline calls this twenty-year memory gap "The Mother," a part who was created to be a mother, and who bore five children in six years and a sixth child eight years later. By the time full consciousness of motherhood came to the part of Caroline's mind speaking with me, her youngest child was fifteen and her oldest twenty-nine.

Caroline's memory structure allows her to remember the addresses and houses where she lived, down to the wallpaper and other details, but not her children as they grew up. That memory remains with the still inaccessible Mother. Caroline, as the current host and mother, is disturbed by the former mother's elusiveness. When I asked Caroline to name any one negative effect of having parts that stood out in her mind, she said, "you don't have access to all the information of your life" and spoke of her ignorance about her own children and her efforts, through therapy, to remember her blank years as a mother. "This particular time is really troubling because we can't access The Mother, can't get the information." Therefore, when I turned my interview questions to the topic of motherhood, Caroline said, "Anything to do with kids, I'm lost."

Besides therapy, Caroline's personal methods of memory retrieval entail a combination of subterfuge and detective work, sometimes with her own children.

> My kids are all older, and one of them said to me, "Remember that ugly purple prom dress?" I had no clue, [but] that's not that upsetting. I could live without knowing about the ugly purple dress. But the thing that bothers me . . . is that she said to me, "Remember the time I was raped?" And you can't say to your daughter that you don't remember this most traumatic experience for her. That's like saying, "I don't care about you," or "You're not worth me remembering." That's not good. And so I say, "Oh yeah, I remember that. What year was that, exactly?" Then she just [gave me] all the information: "Remember I said it was [our next-door neighbor]? Well it was really so and so that did it." Then she filled me in on all the information. So I did lie a bit to begin with.

With such questions, Caroline is now trying to learn from her children what she was like as a mother. The discovery process, together with her own vague memories, has brought up information she finds surprising. While she was speaking with me, she remembered a time in her life she had not thought of "for years," a time when Terry, the part who likes sexual power, and The Mother were "the only two around," an interesting duo. Because of Terry, when Caroline's children were babies, men were "calling and coming over." Caroline thinks these visits took place at night, when her children were upstairs asleep. Some years later, such visits were evidently still occurring, and Caroline does not know what her children might have heard or seen.

Through a chance encounter at the supermarket, Caroline gradually discovered that her daughter, Sally, had seen a counselor for problems at school.

> In the supermarket, [a woman] said, "Oh, hi! How are you doing? How's Sally?" I have no clue who this woman is, none at all. . . . So we're talk-

ing, and then all of a sudden from inside I get an image of this woman being a counselor, like a guidance counselor. I don't know where it came from. And she asks how Sally's doing, and this and that. It's a guess on my part, that that's who she is. And then she mentions a couple of times that Sally had a hard time about certain things. And how is everything working out for her in her life now. So, then what I have to do is go home and the next time I talk to Sally, say, "I ran into so and so. What did she do exactly? When did you know her?" And then she'd go into, "Oh, remember she used to work at the Teen Center," which was a place for teens to drop in and talk to people. So then I'd get all this information.

Years later, Sally went to a detoxification center before Caroline knew that Sally was alcoholic even though the two women were living in the same apartment building. Caroline thinks that because this happened during the tax season, the part called Working Woman had control most of the time and, through long working hours and intense concentration, missed any signs of addiction her daughter may have shown.

Three of Caroline's five sons were sexually abused by a camp counselor, and her daughter was once molested and once raped during the years that Caroline cannot remember, incidents that came to light years later. When the camp counselor was brought to trial, Caroline was asked if she had noticed any changes in her sons' behaviors. To her discomfort, she had to say she did not remember those years and tried, in vain, to explain her amnesia to a lawyer.

The Mother part of Caroline's mind, who began her control with Caroline's first child, departed abruptly. The catalyst for her leaving was a group therapy session at the rehabilitation center where her daughter was undergoing alcohol detoxification. Patients and families were supposed to speak about themselves and their problems. This, evidently, was too much for The Mother.

It was like that was the breaking point for her where [she thought], "I can't deal with this anymore; I'm out of here." Because we came back,

Pam and Jessica; we can remember coming back on that day. That was
the last we ever saw of her. She's gone.

Concerned as she is about her motherhood memory gap, Caroline seeks
reassurance through her children's behavior, encouraged by their continuous attachment to her.

> We don't know what The Mother was like with the children. I don't
> believe . . . I mean, they seem to be fine. Nobody wants to leave me:
> one son lives next door, two sons are still with me. One just moved
> across town. The only one that left was Sally, but she's on the phone
> every other day [and] wants to come back and live upstairs at my house.
> There's something powerful that's drawing them, so I guess we couldn't
> have done all that bad a job.

Nonetheless, Caroline still worries about those missing years. "I don't
have that information, so *that's* bothering me." She fears that her remembered episodes of depression may have deprived her children of empathy,
and that her love was insufficient. "I don't think we could have had [a]
whole connection with the kids. I think we would have shut that down
because we wouldn't have wanted to get hurt by loving anybody that much."
She worries that her own insecurities and lack of knowledge about higher
education held her children back from college.

> We don't know about college, about the different degrees, and we appar-
> ently never thought that was a priority for them. "What do you mean
> you don't know about it, you're fifty-seven years old," you know? But
> we never had that experience; it's something we were never taught. We
> never had anyone that cared about us enough to think [about] that.

When she should have guided her children, she fears she may have failed
from "not knowing how to do things right." She wonders whether The
Mother's protection was adequate, whether her children's sexual abuse could
have been avoided, or if not, whether she, as the mother she is today, might

have noticed signs of their distress. All these uncertainties plague Caroline and make her memory gaps the more frustrating.

Finally, might The Mother part have abused or occasionally been too harsh with the children? She suspects that one child occasionally drove her "over the edge," and a family member's chance remark makes Caroline think that she used to lock her daughter out of the house. More than this she does not know.

Reactions to Caroline's Diagnosis: "They Just Know Me as Me"

Around the time that Pam, Jessica, and perhaps other parts of Caroline's mind regained control of consciousness, Caroline sought therapy and eventually realized that her experiences have a name. She tried to explain the diagnosis of dissociative identity disorder to her children, with mixed results. The child who has always been closest to her immediately wanted to know more about her experiences so that he could understand the diagnosis. He went on a car trip with Caroline, evidently with the express purpose of having her to himself so that he could talk with her about it. Her daughter, Sally, was at first reluctant to hear much about her mother's new knowledge and did not understand why her mother could not remember so many of their experiences together. When Sally would ask her mother, "Do you remember when . . . ?" her sister-in-law would have to remind her, "She wasn't around then; this is somebody else." This is a disturbing statement to have to make to a daughter who perceives her mother as no different from the mother she has always known. Another of Caroline's sons showed little interest and obviously misunderstands his mother's situation. About six months after Caroline's disclosure to him, he saw her at the computer on a chat line she had created for people who have dissociated parts. His comment was, "Oh, are you still doing that multiple thing?" "He doesn't get it," Caroline says, resignedly. Apparently, none of her other sons understands it either. "They're not really interested," Caroline says. "I mean, they just know me as me, and they're happy with that."

For those of her children and their spouses who do understand, the diagnosis has helped them make sense of some of Caroline's puzzling behaviors. When Caroline interrogates the entire household to find out who ate her missing ice cream bar, all can laugh together when Caroline finally realizes that she ate it herself while another part was in control. The diagnosis allows humor to relieve the atmosphere and pull the family together. Her daughter, Sally, also now understands that Caroline does not remember everything she pretends to remember, including the time when Sally was raped.

> Sally said, "You really didn't remember that, did you?" And I said, "No."
> But it was okay for her to say that. I figured I was there when she needed
> to talk about it that night. If I had burst her bubble at that point and
> said, "No, I don't remember this," she wouldn't have got the benefit of
> the conversation that we did end up having.

Also, her children's comments continue to teach her about the mother she once was. Caroline, who now only occasionally drinks wine, came home one day and announced to her daughter, who was sitting in the yard, "I have the most incredible urge to have a glass of wine." To Caroline's surprise, her daughter exclaimed, "Oh no! not my teenage mother coming back." When Caroline asked her what she meant, Sally said, "You used to drink that every single night, . . . don't even tell me she's coming back," uncovering yet another aspect of her former life Caroline, as the current host, knows little or nothing about.

In a way, Caroline is now making up as a grandmother for her lost years as a mother. She "feels like a little kid" when she is with her grandchildren, thanks partly to a nine-year-old part called Vicky. Caroline's house is full of toys, and her grandchildren and their friends play with Caroline and with each other. Caroline speaks of such times with the vocabulary and excitement worthy of the young Vicky:

> We have all these ongoing different games, goofy stuff. We'll have a
> sleepover and rent some scary movies and go to Stop and Shop and load

up on junk food and stuff. We like to do nutty things with them because Vicky's enjoying it all too. I know when Vicky [is influencing me] because it feels good: we feel silly and we feel like a little kid, just like, "I'm going to do cool stuff; it's going to be awesome."

Caroline thinks that when their friends are around, her grandchildren are occasionally mortified at first by her childlike behavior, but then succumb to the general fun of it all. Some of her younger grandchildren have learned from their parents about Caroline's diagnosis. They are unlikely to understand it, and Caroline has never discussed it with them. However, their knowledge, combined with a fifty-seven-year-old woman's unusual ability to be "on the same level" as a youngster, has prompted some of her grandchildren to occasionally ask, "Nanna, has you taken your medication?" even though she takes none. "They just think that I'm whacky sometimes," Caroline says. Even her grandchildren's friends seem to notice that Caroline is unusually good company, as grandmothers go. Caroline happily reported one such friend's opinion, "You're really a lot different than my grandmother. My grandmother doesn't do anything fun."

Caroline perceives that her grandchildren trust her and confide in her as in a good friend. She, in her turn, pours out all her love, pleased that she can now feel such love and knows how to make her grandchildren happy.

> [With] my grandchildren there's so much love there and such a connection with all of them. They're all great kids, and they all love me to death, you know? They're always around me, or calling me on the phone. I love the connection, and hope I never lose that. . . . There [used to be] different parts that would not have allowed us to feel all this love. That just wasn't a possibility for us. Now it is—and it's awesome.

Because of therapy, Caroline now has access to more of her feelings. Although she is none too pleased about some of the feelings she now must tolerate, she thanks such access for her newfound ability, in her late fifties, to love her offspring without fear and remember it.

COMOTHERS AND INCONSISTENCIES

They don't know what they're allowed to do.

—*Samantha*

I'm five foot two; overweight—not horribly overweight, but overweight; I have glasses [and] short, curly brown hair. I'm good with kids. And I think that's about it.

This is how Samantha, a forty-three-year-old mother of eight and stepmother of four, described herself when I asked her to tell me about the parts of her mind. Samantha's mind has separate parts for almost every aspect of her life, including intellectual activities (The Smart One); sex and conversation related to the body (Cecelia); making people like her (Julia); feeling anger (Madelyn); feeling physical and emotional pain (The One Who Feels the Pain); urinating and defecating (Mandy); and more. Samantha, as a part of the host, is "good with kids," caregiving being one of the few aspects of her life she retains under her conscious control. Five of her children are still at home; the rest are grown.

Samantha considers herself suited to her job. She has problems with the older of her four stepchildren, but sees her relationship with most of her children as positive and close.

I can talk to them about anything, and they're pretty open to talking to me about anything. I'm pretty easygoing, but I have my limits, and they know that if they've hit a limit they're not going to win. But they don't hit limits all that often. . . . I think they love me. I love them.

Samantha's description of herself and all that she told me about her behavior with her children suggest that she is a loving, accessible mother who disciplines with restraint. She considers her own main drawback as a parent to be her reticence when her children reach eight or nine years of age and sometimes crave physical affection. "It becomes awkward," she says, but she makes an effort to overcome her reluctance, perhaps simultaneously overcoming memory traces of parental physical contact grossly distorted when she was that age.

Another intermittent drawback is Samantha's self-perceived youth. Now in her early forties, Samantha thinks that she is sixteen, the age at which she became engaged to be married and her father stopped abusing her. When I asked her why she thought she was sixteen, she said she did not know, "but it's starting to not make sense because I have gray hairs." Twice she mentioned the frustration she periodically, but briefly, feels at being such a (psychologically) young mother.

> It's frustrating sometimes because you don't feel like you're old enough to have to take care of all these kids, and you feel like they're older than you are. Sometimes it would feel like I was in high school or middle school and, "What the hell are all these kids doing here? Why am I supposed to take care of all these kids?" It wasn't that I didn't know who they were, it was just their existence seemed incongruous. It was a feeling of, "How can I have all these kids when I'm not even out of high school?"

Such feelings tend to come when Samantha becomes almost overwhelmed by her busy life's duties.

The awkwardness of physical affection and the feeling of being a teenager are comparatively minor problems. A greater complexity comes from the fact that other parts of Samantha's mind share in the responsibility of motherhood. Although the Samantha part is often independently in charge of taking care of her children, two other parts, Julia and The Smart One, both forty-three-year-olds, form a trinity with Samantha for childcare. Julia is loving, and The Smart One is wise, quick, and efficient. All three parts of Samantha's mind are essential to the myriad requirements of motherhood. So interdependent are they as mothers that when one of the children falls ill, for example, The Smart One diagnoses the problem but Julia treats it. All parts who can feel love (namely Samantha, Julia, Megan, Cecelia, Mandy, and Melissa) love the children. The Smart One may not feel love, but she is a comother and sacrificed her career as the best lawyer in her firm in order to keep a shorter work schedule, incompatible with "star lawyer" status.

Samantha had already borne five children by the time she was diagnosed as having DID at age thirty-seven. Before her diagnosis she did not realize she had parts. All she knew was that she heard voices inside her head, her memory sometimes failed her, and motherhood felt like "a roller coaster."

> Sometimes I'd feel all upset about something, and at other times I'd feel not upset. [Or] I'd want to do something with [the kids], and then all of a sudden I wouldn't want to do it. It's hard to know what I was thinking and feeling. . . . Sometimes I'd be really mad about something, and I'd spank one of them or have him sitting in the corner. And then I'd just tell him to get up and go, and I wasn't mad anymore—it was like it disappeared.

Besides these confusing rapid changes in her feelings and wishes, Samantha was sometimes "dropped in the middle of a scene" with her children, having no idea what had just happened or what she was supposed to do.

> A few years ago my two oldest teenagers were fighting, and I wasn't doing the mediating, I guess The Smart One was doing it or Julia. And then all of a sudden I was back and I didn't know what we'd been talking about or whether it had been calmed down—I didn't know where we were in the conflict. I just knew that I had June and Matthew staring at me, and they looked mad, and I didn't know what I was doing. That was really scary. I told them that we needed to take a break for ten minutes. Then I tried to figure out what had been going on. And usually when I worked really hard and tried to remember, somebody [inside] would tell me.

Samantha's part called The Organizer is Samantha's overall memory and controls the switching process. The Organizer generally informs Samantha of what has just happened before she switches Samantha into control of her body. This time, Samantha's highly structured internal organization failed her, and she found herself in the nightmarish situation of suddenly being center stage without knowing her lines. Trying hard to fill in her memory gap, Samantha was rewarded by a prompter's cue, information from another part. Samantha was able to get through this awkward situation without her two children having any notion that their mother's behavior had been alternately governed by two different parts. At the time, even Samantha was not aware that she had dissociated parts. Now Samantha knows who her inner voices belong to and is familiar with their respective jobs and characteristics, including their characteristics as mothers. She can analyze the causes of the roller-coaster aspects of motherhood and try to assess the effects on her children of her emotional and behavioral inconsistencies.

When I asked Samantha if any parts of her mind felt like they were not the children's mother, she replied, "I think the only ones that feel like they're their mother are The Smart One and me and Julia," thus excluding the seventeen other parts, nine of whom are child parts. Samantha's reply illustrates other research showing that for some parents, one or more parts of the mind perceive themselves as unrelated to the children.[8] The other parts of Samantha "just have to be in charge now and then," she says. Samantha thinks that the parts other than the three primary caregivers do not care as much about the children and therefore "let things slide that we wouldn't."

Samantha knows the importance of a parent's consistency in setting limits and in discipline. However, because Samantha must share caregiving with other parts, she sometimes finds consistency impossible. Another part may control only the voice, or the emotions, or the body, rather than taking over completely. Samantha can be furious at a child and want to yell, but the words that come out of her mouth are calm and even. She can want to get out of bed to soothe an upset child but find that she cannot move, not because she feels paralyzed but because another part's will is stronger than hers. She once felt enraged at her two-year-old daughter, although rage is otherwise unknown to her. In this rage, and feeling out of control, she kicked the child's legs several times, an abusive action she told me about with shame, and one that she attributes to a male part called Leslie. She can laugh when her children have drawn with permanent markers all over the freshly painted walls of their room and in retrospect wonder why she was amused rather than furious. She can be angry with a child, then suddenly find that her anger has vanished.

Samantha is well aware of the effects of her occasionally contradictory behavior on her children: "They don't know what they're allowed to do and what they're not allowed to do." When I first asked her in what ways other parts affect her role as mother, her reply was, "I think they make it harder to be consistent; harder to discipline," showing that this problem, shared by other mothers because of their parts,[9] is uppermost in Samantha's mind. Samantha's predicament is like that of any mother who finds that other care-takers such as the child's father, grandmother, or teacher have standards for the child that differ from her own. With Samantha, however, the different standards are parts of her as a whole personality, reflecting her mind's dis-sociated clusters of memories, experiences, and functions. The Smart One, for example, is stricter with the children, careful about what she allows and, in Samantha's view, "overprotective." What happens when Samantha and The Smart One disagree?

> [The Smart One] will tell the kids, "No, you can't have a friend to sleep over," or "No, you can't go to this friend's house," or "You can't go to that party." And then an hour or so later, [the kids] will ask again and I'll say, "Yeah, sure, you can go." And so they get different messages.

When I asked her what it felt like to give her children two such differ-ent responses, she replied,

> I'm glad that I can tell them, "Yes, you can go to the friend's house." It's like a feeling of relief, of "Oh, good, I can say what I want to say." [When I say no,] it makes me feel horrible, 'cause I don't see any rea-

son for saying no, but somebody's saying no. It's very, very frustrating. I mean, I open my mouth, and that's what comes out.

In these conflicts, Samantha has to bear The Smart One's anger at being overruled. "She gets mad at me. She yells at me."

Cecelia, the part responsible for sex, occasionally takes over when the children are involved. Being characteristically fun-loving, the adolescent Cecelia's caretaking standards are different from Samantha's. If the children come in and bother her when she is writing e-mails to men, Cecelia tells them to get out, whereas Samantha would let them stay. While Samantha tells the children to turn off the TV when it is their bedtime, Cecelia lets them watch TV as long as they like. Samantha considers Cecelia "not very good" as a mother.

Cecelia, as the part in charge of any conversation having to do with the body, also takes care of talking with the teenage children about sex. Fortunately, here Cecelia is careful and hypocritical, knowing that it would not be wise to suggest sexual behavior like her own to the children. Also, Cecelia is careful about her own behavior and wears her provocative clothes only when the children are asleep or away from home. If Cecelia followed strictly her own interests and practices in these points, she would recommend unprotected sex with virtual strangers or wear provocative clothing whenever she wished. However, Cecelia loves the children and seems to understand that such advice and behavior could shock and harm them. Here, the strength of motherly protectiveness and/or the need to appear "normal" seem to be paramount, whereas in situations the children could interpret as simply a mother's inconsistency, such as limiting TV time, Cecelia's characteristic leniency prevails.

The part of Samantha's mind called Julia is both more affectionate and somewhat stricter than the part called Samantha. Because her original role in life was to try to make Samantha's parents like her, she now wants Samantha's children to behave in a way that will please Samantha's parents. Also, Julia has stricter standards of cleanliness than Samantha has and wants the children to help her keep the house clean.

Samantha's Children's Reactions: "She Wanted to Know Who Was Her Mother"

None of Samantha's younger children know the reason behind their mother's inconsistent limit-setting, but experience has taught them that a refusal might turn into permission an hour later. They have also learned that they can sometimes manipulate Samantha's moods in their favor. As an example, Samantha described shopping with them: "Oh, look at this cool store, come on, Mom, let's go in this really cool store. Look at this shirt, isn't this neat? Let's go get some chocolate-covered strawberries." By including Samantha in the excitement of being their age, they unwittingly lure Cecelia out, who happily goes into the store and buys chocolate-covered strawberries for all. According to Samantha, the children think they are simply getting their mother into the right mood.

When I first asked Samantha what came to her mind concerning having dissociated identities and being a mother, her response was, "It leaves you more open to being manipulated." She feels this vulnerability acutely, especially when her children use her poor memory to their advantage, declaring, "Oh, I told you about that, you just don't remember." Samantha is repeatedly left in the untenable position of not knowing whether she truly has forgotten or rather was never told.

Some of her children have noticed more than their mother's changes in "mood" and memory. At times, when Samantha is playing with her youngest children, child parts take over her actions and speech although Samantha is also present.

> It's just all of us—I don't know how to explain it. I know they're there because they're the ones who are playing and they're the ones talking to the kids. And every now and then I'll have to interrupt and say something different.

Her voice changes to a child's voice, but her children seem to take no special notice, evidently thinking the change part of their mother's play. At these times, all parts of her mind cooperate so that their participation is subtle enough not to alarm the children, another instance in which protecting the children seems to override individual parts' needs. However, when Samantha is by herself and the requirements of motherhood are in abeyance, she occasionally sits on the floor and plays with toys, fully controlled by the needs of child parts. She remembers that once one of her teenage sons chanced upon her play, laughed, and passed by. Samantha does not know what he thought of this unusual sight.

After Samantha learned her diagnosis, she disclosed it to her oldest child, June, who is twenty-three, married, and lives in her own home. During a time when June was calling her mother more often and spending more time with her, she began noticing behaviors that astonished her. Calling Samantha once at night, June caught her obviously drunk, an entirely unexpected discovery that upset June. Then, during a visit, June used Samantha's computer and discovered Cecelia's e-mails soliciting men. When June asked Samantha about the letters, Samantha claimed that she had not been aware of them, not knowing what else to say.

Finally, one evening, Cecelia's plans proved stronger than motherhood, an instinct weakened, perhaps, because June was by then a grown, independent woman. June saw her conservative, traditional, flat-shoed mother leaving the house wearing high heels and a transparent top with no bra. Confused and upset, June tried to reach Samantha's therapist to find out why her mother was behaving so strangely. At her therapist's suggestion, Samantha disclosed her condition to June, who found the information frightening and confusing. She wanted to know who the parts were and what they did. Samantha said that June also asked a specific question: "She wanted to know who was her mother." Although Samantha as mother is mainly the trio of Samantha, Julia, and The Smart One, she modified the truth to soften the shock to June: "I guess I kind of lied to her. I told her we all were [her mother] and that we'd all taken care of her and loved her and she was everybody's daughter, because that was what she wanted to hear." Samantha felt that even as a grown woman, June would be hurt to learn that some other parts of her mother's mind did not consider her their daughter.

Samantha then told two more of her older children. Assuming that they would otherwise hear the news from June, Samantha preferred that they hear it from her. As far as Samantha can tell, the information makes no difference to them. "It's kind of a 'so what?'" Samantha says, illustrating, like Caroline, the vast difference in children's responses to a parent's disclosure. Perhaps because seeing Cecelia in action made the diagnosis more real to her, June seems to understand it in a way the other two children do not. June even makes practical use of her knowledge. When Samantha and June are talking, June sometimes asks, "Who am I talking to?" If she knows that the part of her mother's mind speaking with her is not a good source of the information she needs, she will ask to speak with another part.

> Like, right now she's expecting my second grandchild. And she'll call and have questions. If she's got the wrong person, she figures it out and says, "Okay, give me The One Who Feels the Pain or Julia or Samantha." [She asks for The One Who Feels the Pain] because she's scared about labor. She's a chicken—I don't blame her.

Samantha has told none of her other nine children, even though two more are in their early twenties, because she thinks the knowledge would simply frighten them and that they would be unable to discuss it and to find out more about it on their own. She also seems to fear that they might turn away from her if they knew. Samantha told June under duress, but also because she felt more confident that she would not lose June's affection as a result. "I told June first because I felt like I had a closer relationship with her and she wouldn't freak out and not love me anymore."

Samantha's way of speaking about her children and the examples she gives of her mothering suggest that her children's welfare is paramount. Yet, the myriad effects of the abuse she endured as a child have taken a toll on her children. Having parts has meant inconsistent parenting, an incident of physical abuse, and fears about what she might have done when not conscious of her body's actions. At various periods of her life as a mother, Samantha has also periodically been too depressed to clean the house; had no food; and precipitously taken her children and left home, chaotic circumstances for herself and her children. Samantha does not know if the children overheard any of the "sex parties" Samantha's first husband held, during which he sold Samantha's body to his friends. The children have also had to experience their mother's repeated two-week hospitalizations, one two-month hospitalization, and several suicide attempts. Samantha recalls that her children were all "real upset" when she had a stillborn child and became suicidal, and that after learning her mother's diagnosis, June asked her which of her other parts had been trying to kill Samantha.

Samantha as a whole personality has parenting parts with motherly love in abundance and her nonparenting parts usually blend in unnoticeably or keep quiet. Yet, Samantha also contends with all those aspects of DID inimical to good parenting:

- Nonloving, nonparenting parts, who occasionally control the mind when children are present, one of whom is rageful

- Different standards of limit-setting among parenting identities

- Short-term memory loss about being a mother

- Self-injury, depression, alcoholism, and suicidality

In spite of her efforts, Samantha cannot help the fact that some effects of her childhood abuse have also affected the second generation.

THE SOLE PART FOR MOTHERHOOD

I was a little peculiar at times.

—*Ellie*

Forty-three-year-old Ellie, as the host, is the only part of her mind responsible for her two children, and she has no large memory gaps in her parenting years. She illustrates that it is possible to be a mother and have a mind in parts but only rarely experience effects of DID that are detrimental to parenting. Other parts of Ellie's mind are in control less frequently than Caroline's or Samantha's, and Ellie has no overtly antagonistic identity. These differences are in Ellie's favor. Yet, Ellie's motherhood does mimic that of the two other women in a subdued form: she has discovered memory gaps of herself as a parent; she has learned that another part at least once used a method of physical punishment that horrifies Ellie; and she is learning from her daughter other surprising things about herself as a mother.

Ellie thinks that a part called Edna, who acts as Ellie's "voice of reason," has helped Ellie be a parent. "I think probably Edna has been the most influential in terms of how I live my life now. She's helped me be a good mother and a good grandmother and things like that." Yet, even as she told me this, Ellie winced. When I asked if Edna had just said something to Ellie, she replied, "No, I was thinking about when I wasn't such a good mother." In spite of the relative smoothness of her parenting years as far as the other parts are concerned, Ellie has regrets as a mother. Thinking back on her own childhood, Ellie remembers a time when she was too depressed and lethargic to speak or to eat more than a few mouthfuls of food. When her weight had dropped to eighty-five pounds, her mother's sole remark was, "I wish to God you'd cheer up." Ellie's daughter once began to show similar signs of distress.

> When my daughter came home with those warning signs I knew that there was something wrong. It wasn't anything like what I had gone through, but she was feeling abandoned and unloved. I hadn't gone through therapy, but looking back on it now, I can see what the problem was: I wasn't there emotionally for her.

Ellie realizes that her episodes of depression, self-injury, and suicide attempts were robbing her children of the love, security, and empathy they needed. These episodes were not controlled by other parts, but other parts' voices telling Ellie their memories sometimes provoked such reactions. Ellie blames herself for having had children before therapy gave her more insight into herself. Forgiving herself for her children's suffering is the most difficult step in recovery, Ellie says, describing her knowledge of her own poor parenting as "the hurt that never heals."

When Ellie was diagnosed at age thirty-eight, both her children were in their mid teens. Ellie did not immediately disclose her diagnosis to her family, fearing to tell anyone because of the stigma attached. "Also, I was afraid of not being believed and that they would think that that was just me being crazy." During this time, flashbacks of childhood abuse memories made Ellie suicidal, whereupon a part called Edna would call the therapist and leave her own name rather than Ellie's. Confusion would ensue when her therapist's answering service would return the call and one of the children would answer the phone. "There's no Edna here," they would say, surprised that their mother would then take the call. "They just thought it was weird," Ellie said, "like, 'Why are you calling yourself Edna, Ma?'"

Effects of Disclosure on the Family: "Maybe That's Why You Used to Have That Scary Voice"

When Ellie did disclose to her children, she told them that dissociative identity disorder was the first diagnosis she had received that made sense to her and that put pieces of a puzzle together. When she explained what the diagnosis meant, her children's immediate response was the familiar one, "You mean like Sybil?" Ellie says that her son was, and remains, noncommittal. "Basically his comment is, 'I'm glad you've found a diagnosis that's comfortable for you.' He didn't say he believed it or didn't believe it." Ellie, who calls her parts "alters," later told her children why she received calls for someone called Edna. "I explained to them after I knew *how* to talk to them about it: 'That was just one of the alters; she was looking out for me.'" Her son's response was, "Well, I'm glad she's looking out for you." Although he is noncommittal, Ellie sees her son as a quietly supportive presence in her life.

One of her daughter Pat's responses to Ellie's disclosure was, "Maybe that's why you used to have that scary voice," making Ellie wonder whether

her voice used to change without her realizing it, as it occasionally still does when Ellie is with her husband. Later on, Pat took a book on DID from Ellie's bookshelf and read it, quietly showing her interest in learning more about her mother.

Otherwise, neither child wants to be reminded of Ellie's condition, and it is not a topic often discussed in the family. However, Pat does seem to realize that the diagnosis explains some of her mother's past behavior, including an episode of physical punishment Ellie cannot remember.

> She said that I had spanked her with a ruler. I felt absolutely *horrible* that I had done something like that. I said I was sorry and that I didn't remember it. And she said, "It was you; I know it was you; it wasn't Dad."

When Ellie explained that "maybe it was one of the other ones," Pat countered, "Well, that's okay—but I *know* it was your hand," revealing her misconception about the nature of having parts and her refusal to exonerate her mother from all blame.

Only once does Ellie remember that her behavior embarrassed her daughter, an incident that occurred at work:

> My daughter and one of her friends worked at [a retail store] with me. And at work one time we got a shipment in. It was in a huge box filled with Styrofoam peanuts. We had emptied the box, and it was still full of peanuts, but I fit very easily into it. I crept into it, [spilling] peanuts all around. And my daughter was a little bit embarrassed. She went, "Get out of the box." [Her friend] was going, "Your mother's so much fun! My mother would never do that!" Pat goes, "Yeah, but your mother's not *crazy*." So I got out of the box on that note.

When I asked Ellie how she felt about her daughter's remark, she first said, "It was okay," then, "It kind of stung a little bit." Like Caroline's grandchildren who are embarrassed by her behavior in front of their friends, Ellie causes a daughter's embarrassment in a friend's presence when playful child parts maneuver an adult's body into age-inappropriate behavior. Her daughter's use of the disparaging term "crazy" also suggests that for all her understanding, Pat is sometimes ashamed of having a mother who has parts.

Now that her family knows the diagnosis, they are able to call Ellie back to control her mind if another part is disruptive or inappropriate. This rarely happens except when a three-year-old part called Jesse needs to play. Even then, within the immediate family, Jesse's playtime is generally not prevented, and Ellie is not embarrassed about playing with toys in front of a family member. "It's better to just let her play," Ellie says, "she's not hurting anybody."

Ellie finds that the child parts are still sometimes helpful because they subtly let her know how to play with her granddaughter. Ellie does not even hear their voices, "it's just knowing what to do." Like Caroline, Ellie uses her mind's access to youthful playfulness to her own and her grandchild's benefit.

Ellie now lovingly helps care for her granddaughter, who lives with her mother in Ellie's house. With her granddaughter, Ellie experiences only those aspects of DID that can be beneficial to parenting: a wise, adult part, and child parts who do not upset children and who know how children like to play. With the aid of her wise helper, her child parts, and her insight into herself and her past, Ellie is better equipped than ever to be a loving, responsive, and responsible caregiver.

> Getting all these memories of what [my parts] went through has certainly affected how I deal with children now, especially with this little one [indicating her infant granddaughter whom she had brought with her to the interview]. Oh God! Can you imagine doing that to a little baby?

I told Ellie my impression that without the diagnosis—made by chance when she saw a therapist because of migraine headaches—she and her family could have gone through life without realizing anything about her parts. She responded to my observation with her characteristic humor:

[We would have thought] that I was a little peculiar at times, eccentric. Only I don't have enough money to be eccentric. You have to be rich to be eccentric. Everyone else is just crazy. [We both laugh.]

THE DIFFERENT TRUTHS ABOUT MOTHERHOOD WITH PARTS

Caroline's, Samantha's, and Ellie's experiences of parenting are dictated by their parts' characteristics, their internal organization and cooperation, and by the memory structures they represent. Each of the three women illustrates a different truth about being a mother who has DID. Like Ellie, a mature, long-standing host can be the mother of her children and be in charge almost as much as a woman who has a unified personality. If she is a good parent, her control helps to minimize any effects of irresponsible or abusive parts or inconsistencies among parts. On the other hand, the host who acts as parent may consist of several parts like Samantha's trio of Samantha, The Smart One, and Julia. One part of the host may be unconscious during minutes or hours of mothering. Or, part of the host may be conscious for events and remember them but often find her behavior with her children influenced by other parts who control her speech, actions, or feelings, separately or together, while she helplessly watches or listens to her own inconsistencies or abusive acts. The same can hold true if the host consists of only one part of the mind. In addition, like Caroline, all consciousness of motherhood can fail a part entirely for years. When that part regains control as the mother and host, she wonders what kind of mothering her children had in the past.

In spite of all their differences in internal structures for motherhood, I found some commonalities among Caroline, Samantha, Ellie, and the other child caretakers I interviewed: Elizabeth has her own two daughters; Reba helps raise her niece and nephew; and for seven years Lucy was a stepmother to her partner's two children. Uncertainty and unease about the effects their problems might have had on their children characterize most of these care-takers. Four of these six women find memory lapses a cause of concern or distress. What happened during the lapse? Was I overly strict or even abusive? Did I adequately protect my child? Did I recently promise something to a child? Did the child confide in me something I should have remembered? Being a mother, difficult enough in itself, is made more so by such unanswered questions. These women's concerns about memory lapses relate partly to the unique difficulties they pose to responsible child-rearing: behaving consistently toward a child, knowing when a child needs soothing, protection, or help, and being sure a child's account of past words or actions is true.

However, "Was I abusive?" is the most pressing question for these mothers, given the childhoods they had to endure and the rage often confined within other parts of their minds. Caroline and Samantha mentioned anxiety about possible unremembered physical or emotional abuse, being the two caregivers whose memories as mothers are most affected. Three of the four biological mothers now know of episodes with a child that shock them. Each of the three either remembers or was told of an abusive action or situation: kicking, spanking with a ruler, shaking a child in rage, and emotional neglect, and each mother is horrified and ashamed of her behavior. One can appreciate the lifelong remorse a loving mother feels on realizing that another part of the mind has harmed her child.

For a fourth caregiver, Lucy, the potential for abuse became a catalyst for prevention. Lucy once had a strange feeling while sitting with her stepson, a feeling recounted by the part of her mind called Rose.

> There was a time we got really confused with boundaries. It was weird. We were sitting [with him], and we all of a sudden went, "Uh-oh, something's wrong." It was kind of like a déjà vu moment: you remember something that happened to you like that. And we didn't want it to happen to him. We had to pull away from the kid because we were really not sure what was going on. We knew if we acted on what the body was feeling, we'd be in trouble.

Lucy may have felt the urge to repeat as a perpetrator the sexual abuse she had experienced as a victim. This revision of the past to gain a feeling of mastery rather than helplessness is well known among formerly abused adults.[10] Conversely, one of her young parts may have considered herself unrelated to Lucy's stepson or to Lucy and therefore free to seduce this attractive, available boy, an experience some mothers have that leads them to unwitting incestual abuse.[11] So shocked was Lucy at this episode of physical temptation that she distanced herself somewhat from the child for a year. Then, for a while, whenever Lucy was with the boy, she "shut down so nobody [got] out," and an emotionally numb part called Nada, "the robot one," took over. This switch may have diminished Lucy's empathy and responsiveness, but it secured the boy's physical safety. As far as Lucy knows, her stepson noticed no difference in her behavior, and as he grew older, Lucy found herself free of any such temptation.

Similar to Lucy, all the women I interviewed who abused a child know or suspect that another part's passive influence over the voice and/or body or a complete switch caused the abusive incident. Samantha and Caroline continue to worry about possible unremembered physical or emotional abuse. Some of their uncertainty may last a lifetime unless they eventually feel comfortable asking their children directly or in general conversations about the family's past.

Four out of these six women's children are also suspected or known to have suffered in other ways from their mothers' DID or other signs of distress. Samantha, Ellie, and Elizabeth used to cut and burn themselves, leaving scars difficult and, for Ellie, sometimes impossible to hide from their children. All four biological mothers know or suspect that, at times, they physically or emotionally neglected their children or were unable to protect them from harm. Depression, suffered by all four women, was the main cause of neglect, and suicide-related hospitalizations or another part's control of decisions caused the lack of protection. Other signs of psychiatric distress such as alcoholism, depression, eating disorders, phobias, and suicidal tendencies are evidently common problems that affect parenting among people who have DID.[12]

These same four mothers each have one or more children who had or still have diagnosable problems, including depression, anorexia, ADHD, and alcoholism. Their children's suffering is apparently the norm rather than the exception. One study shows that the incidence of a diagnosable psychiatric problem is nine times greater among the children of parents who have DID than among children whose parents do not.[13] This high incidence may have complex origins, including a history of mental illness in either parent's family and the child's experiences at home. Those home experiences can include some my interviewees did not mention such as a parent's difficulty focusing on a child's needs due to the confusion of inner voices, or a habit of secrecy and fear that precludes meetings with a child's teachers and the parents of a child's friends.[14] Because children of a parent who has DID can be exposed to so many of the parent's struggles, some clinicians recommend that the children be routinely assessed and helped by specialists in child psychiatry and/or child psychotherapy.[15] Help for the children might coincide with a therapist's work with the parent on possible behaviors inimical to good parenting and guidance toward healthy parenting practices.

The commonalities I found among the women I interviewed correspond with the conclusions of the one study I could locate that highlights the variety of competencies among mothers with DID. This was a study of seventy-five mothers diagnosed with DID.[16] Twenty-nine of those women were found to be "competent or exceptional" mothers. These mothers were defined as those who did all their parenting in one identity or who employed one or more of the following strategies for smooth caregiving: the parenting parts were co-conscious; they shared information; or they collaborated to mobilize their parenting skills. As long as the children were deeply loved and never mistreated, a parent was still considered competent even if her parts exposed the children to inconsistencies.

Thirty-four mothers were considered "compromised or impaired," meaning mothers who were psychologically abusive and also those whose symptoms of DID consistently and intrusively interfered with parenting despite the mother's best efforts. A number of such problems were caused directly by parts, such as a mother assigning adult responsibilities to her child because the part in charge at the time refused those responsibilities; neglecting a child's needs because an inappropriate part was in charge at the time; or refusing to be a parent and abandoning the family. Other problems appeared to be the result of other signs of emotional distress such as depression, emotional numbness, or extensive hospitalizations. Most of the "compromised or impaired" mothers were distressed by their parental inadequacies.

Finally, twelve of the seventy-five mothers were "grossly abusive," physically injuring and sexually abusing their children or placing them at risk. In most cases, such abuse was perpetrated by a part who identified with one of the mother's childhood abusers. Such a part would be similar to Samantha's part called Leslie, who identifies with Samantha's abusive first husband. Samantha attributes to Leslie the one episode she can recall of physically abusing a child.

Like the "competent or exceptional" mothers in that study, all the women I interviewed who are child caretakers love their children and are dedicated to their responsibilities as parents. Like the majority of all the mothers in that study, most of my interviewees have experienced possible or known inadequacies as parents and are distressed by them. They share with those mothers and with countless other parents who have DID[17] the same causes of such inadequacies: parts who confuse, neglect, or physically harm the children and depression, emotional numbness, or repeated or extensive hospitalizations. Those who told me of possible or known inadequacies were the four women who are biological mothers: Caroline, Samantha, Ellie, and Elizabeth. Yet, as far as their memories allow them to know, all of them have been nonabusive and responsible parents most of the time. Physical harm appears to be either unknown or the rare exception among all my interviewees who are child caregivers. However, Ellie knows and Caroline suspects that emotional distance from their children caused some harm and may have lasted for years. Together with the majority of the seventy-five mothers, these four women have found that symptoms of their own childhood abuse, including DID, sometimes interfered with parenting despite their best efforts.

Attributes That Encourage Good Parenting

Lucy, a stepmother, and Reba, a comother, mentioned no incidents of inconsistency, neglect, or abuse. Together with Ellie, those two women have the advantage of being the hosts and the sole identities for parenting, with the temporary exception of Lucy's Nada the robot and Reba's child parts who play with and cuddle her niece and nephew. Reba's mothering is the most tranquil of all, and she is the only caregiver with three powerful advantages in her favor: she is the sole identity who acts as mother; she had had skilled therapy for DID before her niece and nephew were born; and (due to therapy) her other parts cooperate with her, coming out with Reba's niece and nephew only when Reba allows them to do so and under Reba's supervision. Also, therapy had helped Reba recognize the effects her parents' behavior had on her.[18] She instinctively feared that her upbringing might have planted abusive tendencies within her and took courses to learn about child development and anger management.

Although Reba has the greatest advantages, all of my interviewees who are child caregivers have some attributes that encourage good parenting. With the exception of Samantha's part called Leslie, all of my interviewees who are child caregivers seem to have parts who generally understand the importance of motherhood. Although some parts may not see themselves as mothers and have varying standards of caregiving, they generally do not sabotage a mother's responsibilities or refuse to take over now and then if required. With few exceptions, the power of maternal love combined with the instinct to appear "normal" override the multidirectional pull of the parts of my interviewees' minds. Lucy's youthful part Rose said as much when speaking of her own and other child parts' self-imposed quiescence in front of Lucy's (The Big One's) stepchildren: "We were very careful around [the kids] that The Big One stayed out, and when the kids went to bed, then we could be out." These child parts sacrificed their own wishes to the requirements of motherhood, a remarkable deed. Further, all seven women who are grandmothers, mothers, stepmothers, or aunts said that some of the other parts help them as caregivers. Six out of the seven women spoke of child parts helping them know how to play with children; two said that their child or adolescent parts enable them to better understand their progeny or to sense when they need help; and three caregivers described mature parts who help them be good parents and grandparents.

Other parts' shared sense of responsibility for caregiving may help the primary parenting part and her children in more than one way. The obvious benefit is to the parental role of competent and loving caregiver. A less obvious advantage lies in the strength of motherhood as a source of meaning and purpose in life. As such, motherhood may act as a unifier for a mind in parts, encouraging improvement in a mother's overall functioning.[19] Ellie has come to see such cooperation and shared information as an act of what she calls "unit preservation." Ellie is referring to the preservation of the mother's life by sharing knowledge to avoid the inner confusion that can cause despair. In other words, other parts of the mind may cooperate, for the children's sake, to avoid the mother part's possible suicide.

In addition, Ellie, Elizabeth, and Reba also find that as caregivers, playing with children allows them to experience moments of truly carefree childhood. Such moments were never possible when they were young, and the experience as adults promotes a sense of release from the past. As Ellie explains, "A childhood is a hard thing to lose and absolutely wonderful to find again." Each opportunity for release may encourage those parts still lingering among the threats of the past to move closer to the relative safety of current everyday life.

Therefore, other parts can help the parenting part(s), and the responsibility of parenting can help unify all parts. Understandably, mothers like Reba, who alone as the host acts as mother, who has insight into her condition and her past, and whose other parts are generally under control, may not wish to rid themselves of their internal, maternal help.

POINTS TO KEEP IN MIND

- Timely, skilled therapy can be crucial in avoiding the aspects of DID and other abuse-related signs of distress that are inimical to good parenting.

- With or without therapy, having one competent part for mothering, or having several for mothering, each of whom cooperates with the others and shares information, provides the greatest advantage to caregiving.

- Some other parts can help the parenting part(s) be a good parent or grandparent, and the responsibility of parenting can help unify the parts.

- Many children of parents with parts show signs of psychological distress in spite of the parents' best wishes and efforts. However, the children's distress is not always directly related to the parents' DID.

- For the parenting part(s), accepting responsibility for having abused a child rather than blaming another part as though she or he were a different person is a painful but useful step toward promoting self-understanding and mental unity.

10

RESOLUTIONS AND HOPES

See, what we realized is nobody understands what it's like to be us unless you is us. And for anybody that's not, it doesn't make sense. But for us it doesn't make sense otherwise. And when we try to figure out how it will be [to be integrated], it will be like dropping us into a country [where] we didn't speak the language or understand anything, and have to learn all over. 'Cause we process information different.

—Rose, a part of the mind of Lucy, a forty-four-year-old
social worker

◉

Before beginning this study, I had assumed that everyone who had parts would strive for a completely unified mind, a state often called *integration*. The previous chapters have illustrated home and workplace experiences that might make a person wish to integrate. Indeed, many people with minds in dissociated parts have integration as a goal. Yet Barbara, my first interviewee, dispelled my assumption that all the women I interviewed would consider integration desirable. By the time I spoke with Lucy months later, I was no longer surprised at her younger part Rose's conclusion that it makes no sense to be integrated, a conclusion with which Lucy, as the adult host, agrees. Indeed, the previous chapters have also illustrated that some women perceive benefits from having parts, benefits they might lose with integration.

LIFE WITHOUT DISSOCIATED PARTS

In the quotation that opens this chapter, Rose puzzles over the relearning she would consider necessary for life with an integrated mind, using the analogy of entering an unfamiliar country.[1] In fact, none of my interviewees could explain to me how a complete and lasting integration feels to them because none had experienced it at the time of the interviews. Instead, I found that most of them had experienced a variety of other permutations among their minds' parts. These changes led to periods of life without parts of the mind for several reasons, some of which I had not heard of before: parts' abrupt and temporary absence, parts' cooperation and quiescence, temporary or fluctuating integration, or partial but stable integration.

Temporary Absences

I asked Lucy, as the adult host, if she thought that she could function without the other parts of her mind. After her immediate "no" she explained by recounting the experience of having all her other parts temporarily out of commission, "everybody got put away." Her part Rose described that state as "not very nice inside. It was too lonely." Lucy and Rose discussed the experience and decided that as long as they all worked together, they did not have to plan for future integration. The state Lucy described was not integration but other parts' temporary absence. Lucy does not know how it would feel if other parts integrated with her, the adult host. Lucy's experience highlights the distinction between previously separated parts being united (integration) and having parts who are temporarily not functioning (temporary absences). Some of Lucy's other parts were once temporarily "asleep" in an interesting case of jet lag. The experience left Lucy realizing that she cannot do without the other parts when they are absent but not integrated.

> We had been in Europe for a couple of weeks. And when we came home, the time change was really hard for me. I couldn't get everybody back

on the time zone; half of them were asleep. I had driven the kids to school for a long time, [but] I couldn't remember where their school was. I couldn't figure out where I was going. I had the most difficult time tracking things. I was a mess, and I realized that it really was hard without having [them].

Samantha, as one of her mind's hosts, has reached the same conclusion. She is periodically frustrated with other parts and wishes to be left alone. Unfortunately, the other parts sometimes take Samantha at her word and say, "Fine; do it yourself," with severe consequences for Samantha who, as a whole personality, is a lawyer.

I had to take care of the kids and go to work and make dinner and do homework—just do everything myself, and I couldn't do it. I couldn't do it. I didn't know what to make for dinner. I'd go to the grocery store and walk up and down the aisles and not be able to pick anything 'cause I had no idea what I wanted or what I was supposed to be doing. I think one week we had the same meal every night 'cause I'd go to the grocery store and I couldn't make any decisions. I'd just buy the same thing I'd bought the night before so that I didn't have to try and make a decision. I wouldn't remember what spices to put in, and things would taste weird, the kids would complain. I went to work, but I didn't know how to do the work. . . . I didn't know what to do. Then I quit work because I couldn't do it. People [inside] weren't cooperating, and it was just too hard to figure out what to do when. [With my kids] it was really hard 'cause I didn't have as much patience as I wanted to have. And I couldn't really be with them 'cause there were too many other things that had to get done.

The "I" who is the Samantha part alone perceives herself as sixteen years old. Her description of life without other parts is much like that of an adolescent suddenly thrown into adult responsibilities. During her other parts' absence, Samantha had to go on disability and enter a day program at the hospital. During that time, other parts became active again. Samantha's conclusion was, "It doesn't work if one person's trying to do everything." She learned other parts' importance and that it is self-destructive to want to be without them. "It was horrible. I learned a lesson." Nowadays, if Samantha neither feels nor hears her other parts she becomes anxious, fearing that they are not paying attention and that they might leave her again to cope with life alone.

Cooperation and Quiescence

Parts can also become quiescent so that the mind mainly functions as one consciousness even though the parts continue to be separate entities. Ellie, a retail manager, characterizes her current situation this way: "It's almost as though we're all one for the times when everything's going smoothly," describing a group functioning in unison, but with each part still present and the child parts still children. This outcome is sometimes called a *resolution.*[2] Ellie described this resolution as a process in which other parts of the mind and the host draw nearer each other. Originally, Ellie, the host, would not be conscious when other parts were in control. She automatically became co-conscious after each of the other parts explained her- or himself to Ellie's therapist. When Ellie would play with toys alone, a child part would be playing while the adult Ellie was a co-conscious observer. Now that all parts of her mind are even closer together, the nature of her child parts' influence has changed.

> It used to be like I'd be sitting behind my eyes and watching [myself] playing with toys. Now it's like I know what I'm doing and I'm playing with [my granddaughter]. But the influence of *how* to play with [my granddaughter] and what [my granddaughter] will like comes from Jesse and Julie Ann and the little ones. And it's not really so much hearing them say anything to me, it's just *knowing* what to do.

Ellie describes how it can feel when separated parts become more unified. Instead of being unconscious or a dissociated observer of a child part at play, Ellie, the adult host, now remains in control but has access to a special insight into her granddaughter and to a childlike playfulness that is increasingly her own.

Ellie specifically stated that having "everything going smoothly" is required for her other parts' quiescence. She knows that during stressful situations, parts who have reached a semi-cohesive state may once again become independent, vocal, and active as the mind reverts to its old method of coping.[3] For this reason, some therapists advocate full integration as an ideal even while acknowledging that it may not suit everyone.[4] Ellie tries to ensure continued quiescence by planning ahead for stressful times, such as a gynecologist's appointment.[5] She arranges that the younger parts obediently stay in their own "room" and do not come out until Ellie leaves the doctor's office and gives them permission.

Ellie's wise adult part called Edna still makes herself heard whenever Ellie behaves in a way Edna considers incorrect or unjust. Otherwise, Ellie perceives her other parts as silent presences, similar to other women's perceptions of their available but quiescent parts as standing in a group and watching, like a family portrait.[6] When I asked Ellie how she knew that her other parts were there if they no longer speak, she gave me this analogy:

> Suppose you were blind and deaf, but when people come into the room, you would sense it. It's that same sort of thing. Sometimes I have to think—I'll stop and I'll go, "Are they all there?" and kind of count them. I guess that's the only way I can describe it—just a presence.

Like women who describe being switched to another part as "sensing that someone is coming up behind you," so Ellie describes sensing her other parts without sight or hearing. When Ellie asks if they are there, each part answers, enabling Ellie to take a roll call of her mind and reassure herself that internally, all is well.

Fluctuating Integrations

In contrast to Samantha's and Lucy's temporary deprivation of parts of their minds, Barbara's, Veronica's, Elizabeth's, and Ellie's internal silences illustrate varying degrees and durations of integration. However, the integration of parts with each other does not necessarily hold for the rest of a person's life. Barbara, a social worker, for example, has repeatedly felt that she, as the adult host, was integrated with all other parts, but each time only temporarily. Each time the inner silence felt odd, but also gave Barbara a new and acceptable sense of identity.

> I've had periods of not hearing them, and it took some getting used to at first; it was strange. But then I realized I had one voice, I had my own—it wasn't like they were gone, it was like they were in me; they were me; I was them. That was reassuring.

As suspicious as she is about the virtues of integration, Barbara has been distressed when the voices returned separate from her own, or has sometimes found that they indicated a renewed split in her mind that required help. Their return, she said, "was not necessarily a healthy thing." Yet she immediately added that she would miss her ability to wall off her consciousness. "If I can be just happy and golden and not be in touch with anything troubling, that's great!"

Veronica, an environmental planner, is also wary of the idea of life with a unified mind. During what may have been a temporary integration, Veronica once glimpsed what a lasting integration might be like for her. After several other parts, whom she calls "people," had integrated, Veronica, as the host, felt that she was what she called "one" for over a year. Although she continued to be capable of facing her life's challenges, the feeling of being one shook her emotionally and existentially.

> I literally—I didn't know who I was. I remember repeatedly wanting to figure out, "Who am I?" I didn't know who the "I" was. And it was terribly lonely because there was all of a sudden this silence. There was no

other talking; there was no other acting. It wasn't until the self-defense classes that one of my kids came out in the instruction class. So with that I was really happy because I had been so lonely for over a year. There've been people with me since.

Veronica twice uses the term "lonely" and twice puzzles over the meaning of the pronoun *I* to illustrate how alien and saddening her other parts' year-long silence was. "I went through a real grieving time," she said. Veronica's loneliness echoes Lucy/Rose's feeling that parts' temporary silences were "too lonely" and Lucy's dislike of the idea of having "nobody to talk to."

Elizabeth, a teacher, who has no qualms about the idea of complete integration, once thought that she was integrated because she no longer heard internal voices. She was disconcerted when she began hearing them again. After one of my interview questions, she remarked,

> It's almost too weird that I'm getting lots of answers at one time. When I start to feel like that and I'm aware of it, it is unsettling at times. That is how I'm feeling today, which then throws me off 'cause I go, "I thought I integrated; did I not?"

Elizabeth's and Barbara's experiences are shared by many people who believe themselves fully integrated only to later notice one or more parts reemerging or discover one or several previously unknown parts.[7] Elizabeth's surprising "lots of answers at one time" came from previously familiar parts that had been temporarily dormant.

Elizabeth was perplexed by her voices' return, but she is not uneasy with their presences now that other parts have learned to adjust their functions to Elizabeth's present circumstances.

> I'm functioning, and if I still have some part that takes care of this or that, okay. Because now I'm all organized, and now I know I am a combination of many different parts. So it's okay; I can feel all right about it.

Elizabeth has learned to see integration as something flexible and repeated. She borrowed from her therapist the image of herself as something like a pond and her other parts as bubbles that now and then leave the pond, then slowly return.

Partial, Stable Integration

Two or more parts of the mind may join together, or one or more other parts may join with the host, acquiring *integration*. Among the women I interviewed, integrations tend to be quiet, peaceful, and logical. Barbara, Lucy, Reba, Veronica, and Caroline have all had such experiences even though none of them considers complete integration a necessary goal. Mainly, their child parts merged when their jobs were done. Lucy's part Rose said that Lucy's integrations were mainly the parts who had "only little memories" and had "got rid" of those memories. Similarly, Caroline said that her child parts are more or less integrated with a still-active child part called Vicki. The children appear to blend smoothly despite varying playtime preferences.

> It's like they had to say what they had to say, and they were happy about things, but they're not separate personalities anymore. They kind of already blended in to be age appropriate. They're all around eight, nine, ten, so anything that Vicki does makes them happy too—except she doesn't want to play with stupid dolls.

Some parts are perceived as dying when their jobs are done, yet their deaths are part of the integration process. Veronica told me that Gabriel, her "gatekeeper," had died. Gabriel was the part who had the most power over the other parts and who protected Veronica, as the host, from their memories. "He needed to die so that I could be released to face that these things happened, be more responsible for myself. He knew when I would be strong enough to know. And his work was done; he didn't need to be a gatekeeper anymore," she explained. Veronica has held burial ceremonies for all her dead parts and described to me her ceremony for Gabriel. When Veronica realized that Gabriel was dying, she also knew that he had a specific wish:

> It wasn't something that I feared. All I knew is that he was dying and he wanted to go to a beach here. I went there, and the whole way there I was crying, crying, crying. Then I went out onto the beach, and I had Gabriel's ashes. He wanted them thrown out on the waters. So I did that and walked around the beach, and actually felt peace and relief.

When I, with my singleton's mind, asked Veronica if she had been holding physical ashes, she sighed, then replied,

> You're kind of talking about reality as others see it and my reality. As far as having his ashes, no. I, the public self, did not see anything in my hands. But I knew I had his ashes. I didn't really think much of it at the time. Looking back on it, I say now "spiritual ashes." But we had merged somehow between his death in the car as we were driving out and my walking onto the beach.

Veronica distinguishes between her perceptions as the host, "I, the public self, did not see anything in my hands," and her inner knowledge, "I knew I had his ashes." She grieves for a part and honors his dying wishes through actions in her reality as well as in the reality that others see. Her use of the passive "we had merged" shows that the integration occurred spontaneously without any conscious facilitation by the host. The part of her mind called Gabriel knew that keeping traumatic memories from Veronica, the host who functions in the world, was no longer beneficial. "He knew when I would be strong enough to know. His work was done."

Like Veronica's, some integrations occur spontaneously, without a therapist's facilitation and without conscious facilitation by the host. Such integrations occur more often among child parts who hold the memory of particular events and have told those memories, rather than among parts who still have a major function in a woman's life.[8] Some women hardly notice integrations that are spontaneous, or realize only after the fact that one or more parts are no longer there. After the age of forty, a person may find that she switches less frequently and that fewer parts seem active than in the person's younger years.[9] Then, as a woman reaches her seventies, she may find that parts have merged spontaneously even if their memories remain inaccessible. Some researchers think that the increased dormancy and atrophy of parts with age could be due to the decline of a person's ability to hypnotize herself in old age.[10]

Reba gave a detailed description of her integration process. She has experienced the most integrations of all my interviewees, having had forty-two parts become only nine. Reba says that although her therapists call these changes integrations, she and other parts call them "joining together." Reba critiqued this chapter and, in awkward, printed letters rather than her usual written hand, inserted this comment from an eight-year-old part called Annie: "I say we *joyn* together cuz it happens when difrent ones of us get better and feel more *joy* than sadness or fear." With this simple sentence, Annie explains when and why some parts of the mind previously frozen in the negative emotions of a child under threat can be ready to integrate with parts who can feel the positive emotions of life in safety.

"It's just happened naturally," Reba said, as parts, mainly the younger ones, told Reba's therapists their memories. Once they released the memories, they "felt like they didn't have to be separate anymore." Reba's words evoke joining together as a willing and peaceful retirement from active duty, with the impetus coming from the parts themselves. "At different times, they just decided they didn't want to be separate anymore, like their job was done," another illustration of a part spontaneously ceasing to be separate once her purpose has been served.

Reba's integrations are a collective experience. When parts say they want to join together, Reba has what she calls an "internal conference." At that conference, together with a therapist, all parts of Reba's mind plan both practically and emotionally for the change. The practical side is vital because parts are like a workforce, with each one having one or more specific responsibilities. Planning for a part's integration is like planning for a worker's departure without rehiring to fill the vacancy. In Reba's case, some of the responsibilities are mundane but essential practicalities: Who will take care of the backyard? Who will keep the car running? Others were in charge of talking and meeting with family members, and Reba and other parts had to decide, "Who's going to be there and how are we going to handle it?" Fortunately, Reba, as the host, is the professional nurse so that no integrations have involved her work.

Just a month before our interview, two parts of Reba's mind, the seven-year-olds Amy and Angie, joined with an eight-year-old called Annie. Their names, ages, and Reba's visual placement of them together on one branch of a tree of parts she drew suggest that each one was a part of related experiences ready to join together to form a new, more cohesive component of Reba's memories. Amy and Angie had long expressed a wish to join with Annie. They would write in Reba's journal that they did not wish to be separate any longer. They even stated that it was "too hard for them to stay separate," as though once they had been relieved of their purpose they had not enough strength to stand on their own. Amy and Angie also wrote that they felt worn out from having been continuously alert and vigilant for years. Once they had released their memories and seen that they were safe from harm, they wanted "to be able to rest" by joining with Annie. Reba illustrates how parts who have been in a constant state of defense against threat finally realize they are safe and long for peace. Reba explained that many of her integrated parts had felt that integrating would allow them to finally rest.

Amy and Angie's wish was delayed because Annie did not want them to "go away," and Reba's therapist said that the integration should be something all agreed on. Reba and all other parts involved in the integration discussed the matter, preparing for the feelings of loss and grief that are often an aftermath of integration.[11]

It was several months of them saying that this is what they wanted to do and talking with Annie about it and helping her feel comfortable with it before they actually did join with her. We would talk about how even though we wouldn't be able to *see* them as individuals anymore, they would still be a part of us, and they and their strengths, and talents, and abilities, and skills, and feelings, and memories, and everything would always stay with us. And that yeah, it would take some time to get used to not having them as individual parts anymore, but that it would be okay because they would still be with us and we'd be stronger together.

Once Annie felt comfortable with this prospect, the integration itself was spontaneous and took place at Reba's home, with Reba's wise part called Helper assisting the process, just as she, the internal matriarch, assists almost all Reba's integrations. For this integration, Reba seemed to use visualization, or "head pictures," as some of my interviewees called their powerful capacity to create or obliterate people and places in their minds. In this case, Reba's mind used the image of squeezing three people together until two of them dissolve into the remaining person.

And then it was just something that happened very naturally. Helper took the three of them in her arms and held them, and we all hugged them and held them for a few minutes. And it's just like the three of them blended together into one, with Annie being the one still separate.

Reba conceded that in spite of careful preparation for the event, the sudden absence of the two parts was painful, especially for Annie, who was upset because she could no longer see them. Yet when she "listened with her heart," as Reba said, Annie could hear and feel them, and eventually felt stronger and happier because the three were now one.

Reba's many integrations have had five preconditions:

1. The part was able to tell what happened to her or him in the past.
2. The therapist believed the part's memory.

3. The part realized that what happened in the past was not the part's fault.
4. The part wanted to integrate.
5. All other parts of the mind, including the host, agreed to the integration.

Other personal narratives and research accounts reinforce the importance of these preconditions.[12]

The wish to join together always came from Reba's other parts themselves, and integrations occurred more quickly among the child parts who felt no urge to continue living separately. Slower integrations occurred when some child parts wanted to grow up before integrating, which they did while Reba watched:

> It was really an interesting process. Two of the male parts, Billy and Tommy, started off as ten-year-olds. And when they started talking about wanting to grow up and be bigger and stronger, it's like inside we could see them growing up to these young men, instead of these little pesky boys. And when they finally decided that they wanted to join with Helper inside of us, they were more like nineteen, twenty years old instead of ten. They were strong, very protective young men that took care of us and kept us safe. And then they decided that they could do the job better if they were joined together with Helper.

Reba's parts decide for themselves whether to remain their same ages or to grow older, and Billy's and Tommy's impetus for growing older and for joining together was to do their jobs as protectors better.

Reba's parts who were always adolescents also needed time to integrate. After they had told their memories, been believed, and felt free of blame, they wanted time to "be themselves" or "have fun." Whereas Reba's younger child parts simply yearned for rest, these older parts wanted first to behave like youngsters once they were unburdened of the terror and guilt of their memories. Then, "eventually they would decide that their job was done,"

Reba said. Here again, "the job" was pivotal in decisions to join together. Those adolescent parts of Reba's mind recognized that they could relax and enjoy themselves, then become parts for appropriate protection in a mainly safe environment.

The process of integration can differ from person to person and from one integration to another in the same person. Reba's process of joining together is often initiated by parts of Reba's mind writing messages in her journal about their wish to integrate. The parts Billy and Tommy, for example, wrote to the part Circle. The message initiated a gathering during which all parts of Reba's mind congregated, talked, and watched the process of three parts becoming one.

> I think we had gone to get ready to go to bed, and we were sitting on the bed, writing in the journal. And it was Circle that they went to first and told her that they were ready to join together with Helper and that's what they wanted to do. Then Circle kind of called a family conference, like, "I know it's late, but we need to have a conference and we need to have it tonight." It wasn't chaotic, it was a peaceful, gentle kind of occurrence and it seemed natural; it just seemed the right thing. It was almost like they stepped into each other and then stepped into her, just kind of a melding together. I could see it happening inside. 'Cause when Billy and Tommy joined with Helper, the rest of us who were still separate were all kind of together at the time, and talking with them, and watching them join together.

Here, Reba seems to be describing an action, a movement within her mind that she could "see happening." Reba looks on at her mind's capacity to fundamentally change, just as it did when dissociated, personified parts first became active during childhood. Her description, so evocative of a family ceremony, echoes some other women who describe one part's merger with another as a ceremony or ritual.[13] These ceremonies may involve gathering or dancing in a circle and are sometimes likened to a wedding, a joining together that ends one phase in life and begins another.[14] In fact, Reba's preferred term "joining together" is reminiscent of the repeated references to the joining of two people within traditional wedding services across Christian denominations.[15]

Although Reba's therapist helps Reba prepare for and process the integration, most integrations take place in the comfort and privacy of Reba's home. One exception was when two parts wanted to join together but "didn't know how to do it." The therapist's instructions to Reba were to relax, close her eyes, call her other parts together, and picture how they wanted to join together. Reba's therapist simply gave suggestions to help Reba's two parts, although some therapists verbally guide their clients through the necessary imagery,[16] taking an active role as facilitators.

When I asked Reba if anything in her life had changed as a result of the integrations, she first said, "I think we've become stronger," then changed the pronoun to the singular, "and I myself have become stronger." Reba now has more of her mind united in the relatively safe reality of her adult life, like the layers of bark on a tree that strengthen the trunk. Because of the integrations, Reba, the adult host, is now responsible for housekeeping, grocery shopping, preparing meals, attending church, paying the bills, and all the daily general duties of life. Rather than simply being the professional taken care of by other parts as soon as she leaves her office, Reba is now more in charge and willingly so. Reba has become "braver," a term her part Annie uses to describe Reba's new self-assertiveness. Reba now stands up to her parents and to other adult family members rather than letting them manipulate her, and she protects her niece, nephew, and other children from her parents. She is also able to help the people with dissociated identities she has met through the Internet, using her experience to assist them during their hard times. Her growing self-confidence in her ability to help herself and others has made all parts of Reba's mind happier.

"WE LIKE THE WAY IT IS"

With so much possibly to gain by having some parts integrate, it might seem logical that Reba, or anyone who has parts, would strive for complete unity of mind. Lucy disagrees with this logic. Speaking with the character-istic forthrightness of her younger part Rose, she challenges the assumption that a unified person knows what is best for someone who has dissociated identities. "Everybody says it's better to be one, but they've never been other than that, so how do they know?" Rose once asked her therapist what advantages Lucy might have in being one unified identity rather than sev-eral. On hearing that unity might give her more energy, Rose replied, "We'd rather have us." *Integration* is a bad word for Rose, who is emphatic about remaining separate and active. Referring to Lucy, Rose says, "*She* gets to be here, so do *we*." Speaking as the adult host, Lucy agrees that in spite of occa-sional drawbacks, she is content with her mind's structure.

> I think that for me it makes sense to be where I am [partly because] I can't—I guess what I realize is I've lived this way and managed for all of my life. And out of the issues that were dysfunctional [and] that I wanted to get away from, this one didn't have the high priority. And I don't view it as dysfunctional, actually. I like the way that I am, and it works.

Some of Lucy's other parts have already integrated, mainly the ones who had "only little memories" and had "got rid" of those memories, Rose said. Lucy has thought about complete integration, but her part Rose asks, "Why would we want to?" Rose explains that the very strangeness of being uni-fied makes it undesirable.

> See, we don't know what that would be like. We don't even know what *we'd* be like. It's kind of an interesting thought. We tried to figure out what it would be like to have nobody else to visit with, and play with, and talk to, and chat. But we couldn't. We've never been that way.

Rose told me that she had read books by people who integrated. "They say it's quiet. And we don't like it quiet; we like the way it is." Stillness means that one is solitary, a state that can be difficult to bear when a person is accustomed to inner company. Rose is not alone in fearing the possible consequences of unification.[17] She would find her concerns supported by the accounts of some women who have largely or completely integrated. Even while praising some aspects of integration, they speak of not knowing how to cope with their newfound emotions, of a husband who feels alienated by his wife's integration, of being disoriented by their new perceptions of themselves and others, and of no longer being able to relate to people.[18] The newly unified person can no longer psychologically escape the troubles and pain of the world. One therapist admits that achieving unification often leaves an adult client afflicted for the first time with "single personality disorder," the array of everyday challenges of life with a unified mind.[19]

"The Gift of Having It"

When I first began interviewing women for this project, I had read about DID only as a problem, and indeed, my research illustrates the disruption and distress it can cause at home and at work. Even when all but one of the women I interviewed spoke of DID's positive as well as negative effects during adulthood, I assumed that all my interviewees would consider DID a liability. After all, they had told me about parts precipitating job resignations, hospitalizations, suicide attempts, and child neglect or maltreatment. They spoke of lowered professional potential, disrupted partnerships, and the necessity of sacrificing motherhood. Having minds in dissociated parts has made these women fear insanity and feel like "freaks." Yet Caroline already illustrated in her first-person account of her working life how wrong my assumption was. Certainly many people feel stronger, more capable, and more at peace when all parts are united. However, I underestimated the sense of gratitude and loyalty some people feel for the parts of their minds who suffered so greatly and shielded the host's consciousness. When Ellie thinks of what a child part went through for other parts of Ellie's mind, tears of pity and gratitude come to her eyes. Ellie knows that the child she cries about is a part of herself as a whole personality. Yet she still perceives the child as another person, a child who sacrificed herself for the adult Ellie's sake.

Reba expressed gratitude with love when she spoke in a tearful voice of the possible changes that would come with further integrations. Although Reba knows that she would probably grow stronger, she would feel a loss if her remaining child parts integrate.

> I am very attached to them. But I know that if it's something that they really want, I can't deny it to them just because I'm emotionally attached to them being separate. I have to do what's best for them, let them grow in the ways that they need to grow, and still always be there to support them. And I don't know how things would change except [that] I would really miss them.

Reba speaks like a mother whose children are leaving home who is reluctant to accept their independence and their absence. Reba refers to her other parts lovingly, pointing out how much she has learned from them and tries to remind herself that these child parts would become a part of her increasingly whole personality. Reba, however, like anyone who faces the loss of beloved people, would miss seeing them and hearing their voices. The idea that someone can miss having an attribute of a "mental illness" was one of the many surprises my interviewees offered me.

Barbara and Caroline referred to complete integration as "killing" other parts of their minds. Other people have spoken of parts "dying" and abandoning a person who still needs them.[20] Parts themselves may fear annihilation, feeling that integration will be the equivalent of death.[21] While talking with me, even the term *integration* seems to have caused a shift in Barbara's consciousness. Just before she used the term, her voice dropped to an almost inaudible level and she whispered, "I don't like that word too much." Later in the interview, when therapy and integration were again the topics, her vocabulary appeared to be influenced by one or more child parts who did not want "that therapy lady" to try to integrate parts of Barbara. "It felt bad," Barbara said. A compromise for Barbara is the idea of partial blending, like the blending of colors. She is comfortable with the idea of red and yellow blending to make orange, as long as a tip of pure red and a tip of pure yellow remain. "So it doesn't mean that Slugger has to go away totally, 'cause he comes in handy."

In addition, as long as all parts generally cooperate, some people simply prefer having separated states of consciousness and even consider them assets. Caroline finds having a compartmentalized mind professionally useful because one part can be responsible for work without having the clutter of other concerns in Caroline's life. Caroline, as the host, enjoys the purity and innocence of having separated memories and functions. "We still need the separateness," she said, explaining that she does not appreciate having to experience painful feelings as part of the package of improvements she has achieved through therapy. "Sometimes it's hard to get other people's feelings. [But] now we can't help it, and I don't like that. I don't like not being able to shut that off." If Caroline knew Barbara, Caroline would probably support Barbara's wish to retain her capacity to shut out the cares of adulthood. Caroline cautiously approves of her therapist's version of a therapeutic goal, a version which could be called *harmonization*[22]: "My therapist [says it's] like an orchestra. Everyone has a different function, and so we all need to do it right to make it sound good. I guess that's a good analogy."

No parts of Barbara's mind had permanently integrated at the time of the interview, and she continues to appreciate them. Because other parts vary from Barbara, the host, in their likes, aptitudes, and ages, Barbara has an internal task force. Because she is now largely in control, she can call on members of her task force and yet remain the adult host. She now perceives her access to such a varied group as an invaluable asset for the requirements of her life, from repairing the vacuum cleaner at home (Chore Boy), to calculating the budget at work (Math Girl). Barbara is not sure she wants to make complete and stable integration a goal:

> I don't know that I need to feel full integration. I resist it in ways because
> if you can separate from the complexities, it's uncontaminated. You can

just *be* someone who likes to have fun. You don't even have to think about work or trouble or chores. You can just be all young, and play, and tell jokes, and eat candy, and that's all that matters. I think everyone should be able to have that without contamination by worries and concerns of paying the bills and all that kind of stuff.

By using the term *contamination*, Barbara illustrates her preference for the ability to occasionally be a child. In fact, she thinks that everyone should be able to experience such pure, fun-loving irresponsibility at times.

Elizabeth has nothing against the idea of complete integration, yet she finds her other parts' degree of quiescent and cooperative separation advantageous. Like Barbara, Elizabeth can retrieve parts that are particularly helpful in specific situations. She described her current internal state:

I like to think of it as changing hats now. Like, if I need to call on the part of me that's more secure and confident in school or business or parenting, I feel like I can call that part of my personality up to take care of that situation. And I feel like that's what I've learned as far as integration goes, to switch hats or switch roles.

Instead of striving for full integration, Elizabeth's current approach is, "If you have it, use it." She enjoys the acute sensibility ("my radar") that her child parts and her past experiences give her.

Elizabeth is one of the women who point out distinct advantages to having dissociated parts. *Advantageous* is certainly not the adjective that would immediately come to mind when thinking about having DID. However, my research shows that when other parts become well known to the host and no longer cause much trouble, the host can find that having them brings special skills, insights, and talents.

For example, keeping other parts reasonably obedient and happy requires skills useful to the host in the outside world. Due to their inner structure, some people with DID have daily practice in negotiation. They know the importance of listening to others' opinions, of discussing important matters with others, and gaining consensus before action is taken. When Barbara feels the pull of her other parts' opposing wishes, she tries to find a compromise on which they can all agree.

> It's like consensus in a way; you have to have consensus or some kind of compromises that are livable. Sometimes it's like an average, "Okay, you would ideally like to be able to do this and you would like to do that. And what's the way that runs along the middle."

Barbara indicated a strong sense of fairness when she compared her consultations with the other parts of her mind to the consultations necessary between two people in a harmonious partnership.

> I think it's important to hear all aspects of myself in terms of making a big decision. These days I do take the time to have a lot of discussion about the pros and cons. If somebody says, "No, definitely not," is that just fear of change, or is that a legitimate thing you want to listen to? Like, if you're used to being in a marriage you're not going to take a vacation without consulting your partner. Whereas if you're single, you just do it. So, I'm just used to being in this kind of thing.

Caroline pointed out that internal negotiation gives her experience for negotiating on the job. She spoke of having learned to "pay attention to other people." When talking about her growing clientele as an accountant for tax services, she said,

> The different personalities working together inside [has] probably got a lot to do with how I work with people outside. Because you learn that. My biggest thing is that you want to treat people the way you want to be treated yourself. That's just how I am. But I think a lot of that came with learning how to manage all of us.

Caroline explained that she manages to live with all parts by being kind, taking all parts' feelings into account, and negotiating with them. Now, Caroline uses those talents to her personal and professional benefit.

Some women also make practical use of their different levels of wisdom and insight. These levels are the adult host, child or adolescent parts, and sometimes a wiser, calmer level, perhaps perceived as an older woman. Child parts, so pitiful because of their memories, so embarrassing when they are unruly, can sometimes be useful when under control. The resources of their youthfulness can be quarried but remain under the host's adult supervision. Caroline and Ellie, both grandmothers, spoke of their capacity to relate to their grandchildren. Both of them understand what their grandchildren like to an extent inaccessible to singletons. In Chapter 9, Caroline related her ability to enjoy and play with her grandchildren on the children's level to a depth unusual in adults. A child part helps her empathize with her grand-children and makes them happy in her company. Both Caroline and Ellie remain in control as the adult hosts but are influenced from the inside by younger parts in what and how to play. Both of them may have much to teach others about how to be enjoyable grandparents.

Child parts' good influences show themselves at the workplace as well, a finding I had definitely not expected. Elizabeth, a teacher in special edu-cation, has child parts who give her ideas for student projects.

> The projects I would come up with for a child or a group that I was working with was because that's what the kids inside me were talking about that they wanted to do. Often it filtered in like that. And it was great for the kids in the room because it was like the same age for a lot of them. But as a teacher there's always that upper level of functioning, being appropriate, taking care of the kids. Yet, there were points in every day that *I* could experience those children inside *me*, playing and grow-ing and learning things they never got to do before.

As Elizabeth explains, the children in her classroom and the child parts of her mind benefit from exposure to each other. Elizabeth seems to have unusually acute perceptions about children. The school principal where

Elizabeth works once remarked on what Elizabeth calls her "sense about a child," an ability to notice things that slip by the other teachers. "Oh, you have such good instincts," the principal said, little knowing the source of Elizabeth's instincts.

Both therapists I interviewed spoke of an unusually strong empathy with their adolescent clients' needs and ways of thinking. Barbara is one who now uses her capacity to feel "little" as an advantage.

> Sometimes it is useful [because] I'm able to relate to our clients more. I'm running a new program that involves children. I was ordering supplies, so I was watching some videos of kids' stuff and [feeling little] made me think certain things and feel certain things better than staying big. Because I was little at the time and I saw a word I didn't understand, I could say, "Wait a minute, this video uses too many big words, people aren't going to understand it. Are you sure they should say 'entitlement'? Do you think they know what that means? Or 'empowerment': that's too big a word; why don't they just say 'feeling good.'" So that helps sometimes. It can bring different perspectives to things, straight from a kid's point of view.

When she and her colleagues make posters to market programs specifically to thirteen-year-olds, Barbara can tell her colleagues which terms to avoid and which to use to attract that age group. For parts of Barbara's mind, her teenage perceptions and cognitive abilities are still present.

> I'll think of ideas from my teenage self, what's going to appeal to them. Some people are out of touch with their teenage years: when you're forty you haven't been a teenager for twenty-one years. You can maybe remember being a teenager, but if you remember it like it was yesterday or like it's today, it's a little fresher.

Lucy, also a therapist, thanks her fragmented mind for a heightened perception of people of all ages. At work, she focuses all parts on her client. "We put everybody to work," as Lucy's part Rose explained,

Yeah, it's like all the little ones we say, 'Okay, get your ears out and all your senses, we're going to listen.' And we figure it out. We read people very well.

Rose said that for friends who are troubled or for clients, Lucy and several other parts "kind of go inside and figure things out." By focusing, Lucy "gets information" about what is on a client's or friend's mind. Other parts send Lucy what they call "pictures" of their perceptions about a client. Lucy confirmed that her perceptions are visual and that she then compares them with the client's words to see if they fit. When she tells the person what she perceives to be the problem, she usually finds her perception confirmed, causing some people to ask, "Are you reading my mind?" Rose says that she does not yet understand how she does this and is cautious about telling others because "it's kind of scary" and some people consider her "nutty" anyway. Later in the interview Lucy, as the adult host, confirmed Rose's description of going inside her mind and getting insights from other parts.

I don't understand the process, but what I do know is when I'm in there, I get more information. I get it from them, and I can tell it's from having them read people or pick up on things. I used to think it's coincidence, but then after having so many people that I've worked with go, "How do you know this?" [about] things that they've tried to hide, it's like, "I guessed, 'cause it just fits," and I can't explain it to them.

As Lucy said, she suspects that her acute perception comes from child or adolescent parts "picking up on things." A child of abusive parents has to try to read her parents' minds to assess their moods and protect herself as best she can. As part of her self-defense over the years, she may develop an unusually acute ability to perceive another person's state of mind. Lucy understands this herself. She explained that she learned to be perceptive as a child because she had to "read people all the time" to assess her own safety. "We've always known how to do that. We could walk into a room and tell who was fighting with who and what's going on. And as a therapist, we do the same."

With part of Lucy's mind still in childhood, she can continue to use the full strength of an abused child's ability to "read" another person's mind. Lucy calls her acute perceptions part of "the gift" that can come from having dissociated parts of the mind.

> Probably the biggest negative has been realizing [that] it happened because of the abuse. And when I don't focus on that, I look at it as the gift of having it: the talents that come from that, and the skills. [I] understand a lot, do a lot, manage a lot, and process pretty quickly [because] there's ones that do different things [and have] different skills and talents.

Like Lucy, Elizabeth calls her acute perceptions about her pupils "a gift." Both women used the term "gift" to mean the same things: the talents, skills, and insights that they otherwise might not have, especially with their child or adolescent clients and students. Elizabeth first heard this term from her therapist, who accurately predicted the change that would come in Elizabeth's attitude about having a mind in parts.

> That's what Gerry always said, and I didn't understand her. She'd say, "It's going to be a gift, it's going to be a treasured gift, Elizabeth." And I'm just like, "Really?" And she says, "Yeah, wait."

In addition, some parts seem to strengthen the host's character. Reba, for example, finds that child parts are role models for her, just as an admirable friend or mentor can be in the outside world. From a ten-year-old, physically disabled part, Reba is learning "patience, and how to be happy in spite of problems." From a happy, vivacious eight-year-old part who used to only cower in fear, Reba, the host, is also learning how to be cheerful, friendly, and loving despite a stifling past.

Similarly, some women learn from a level of mind who acts as the host's wise parent even when the host has herself entered adulthood. Ellie is now a grandmother, yet a part called Edna still acts as Ellie's parent and has soothed and advised Ellie like a parent throughout life.

Edna is the oldest. It's really weird; it's like she's always older than me 'cause she mothered me. I had that mother figure to be my mother. Edna provides nurturing mostly and faith [in God and] in the worth of each person. [S]he was strong when I needed to be strong. It's hard to explain the calming influence that she has brought to the whole unit.

During childhood, the Edna part of Ellie's mind managed to remain sufficiently outside events to act as a calm advisor, much like Reba's "grandma" part called The Helper. Ellie describes Edna as being almost like her conscience, but a conscience with a voice different from Ellie's. The advantage of Edna's different voice is a conscience that insists on being heard. Edna helps Ellie treat people well at work and reminds Ellie at home of "the good things that a grandmother can be." Even now that Ellie is forty-three, Edna plays her parental role. On mornings when Ellie does not want to get up and go to work, Edna's voice is still there to command, "Hey, wake up!"

"I Have to Hide Who I Really Am"

Even as the women I interviewed use their extraordinary minds creatively, they can rarely tell other people about the reason for their unique talents. Some of them evidently hope that my study of their lives will help them out of the loneliness of having to hide who they are. As Caroline said, "There's a lot of times you'd just like to explain yourself and have someone understand what you're explaining, you know?" In a letter, Reba expressed such a hope between the lines when she thanked me for my research, then wrote,

I/we still feel like I/we have to hide our "condition" from everyone except our therapist because of the severe lack of understanding the truth about people with DID. It's a lonely existence—yes, even with multiple persons within, the outer existence is lonely due to not being able to be completely honest with other people about "me."

Many of Reba's parts had already integrated, but she is not eager to have all of them integrate because she would miss them. Nonetheless, her letter to me makes it clear that the inner company of other parts is no substitute for attachments to tangible people. Reba's words reveal that she considers honesty about having parts a prerequisite to close friendships. Barbara agrees, "If someone's an important person in my life and I want there to be an intimate connection, I'm going to risk telling them because if you're holding something back like that you really can't be close."

Some of my interviewees have been conscientiously blocking intimate friendships since adolescence. Gabbi maintained a decided distance from schoolmates from high school onward so that no one could discover "what is really me."

> The more abnormal I felt, the more I felt that people could not under-
> stand. And I felt like I didn't have a whole lot to share with people. You
> know, when people get together as friends, you talk about your past and
> your family and your this and your that, and those are things I never
> wanted to talk about. So there wasn't a whole lot left.

Gabbi now regrets that she did not trust people enough for friendships earlier, saying that having close friends would have helped her healing process.

When I asked Elizabeth about the most important negative effects of having a mind in parts she first said, "I felt crazy for a long time," then added, "It was hard for me to have people really get to know me," which Veronica repeated in almost identical words: "I . . . have this fear of people knowing me." In Chapter 5, Reba and Gabbi both spoke of their enforced isolation from their colleagues for fear that their colleagues might get to know them too well for comfort. "I don't socialize," Gabbi said, speaking of her workplace, "nobody really knows about my life." "I have to hide who I really am," Reba said, echoing other women's words and again using the term "hide" to describe her personal secrecy. Reba avoids chats with colleagues, fearing to reveal too much about herself. "They won't understand, [and I don't want them] to suddenly be afraid of me or not want me around them."

Being active and professional would normally increase a woman's social life and friendships, bringing her in contact with more people and work-related social events. Ironically, being a professional may heighten any loneliness a woman with DID feels. The professional world does not expect such members among its ranks, and professional women with DID do not expect to find others like them at the workplace. Even if they expected to, how would they find them?

Veronica, an environmental planner, said that she has no trust that the business world could accept people who are different, "and I'm in the mainstream corporate world," she said. She twice mentioned her social loneliness and once asked me if there was any way that I could help her get in touch with other women like her who have DID and lead full, responsible lives. Through a support group, she knows a few women who have DID but none who are functioning well. "So they're not really a resource for me other than to be sympathetic. And because of their own circumstances they are not able to do much with me." Reba critiqued two chapters for me and wrote notes about her reactions. She wrote about her amazement at finding how other women's experiences resemble her own, "It's so nice knowing other people are similar to us and we are not all alone in having DID and being what our therapist calls 'high functioning.'" Reba knew that she is not alone in having DID, but was surprised that she is not "all alone" in having DID and being a respected professional.

Many people are friends, colleagues, partners, or relatives of the Rebas, Gabbis, and Veronicas in their communities without realizing that these women have minds in several parts. Women with parts are known and loved as people to whom others can relate, just like anyone else. These women want to be accepted as people with dissociated identities who are contributors to their communities. They want to be appreciated for the gifts of perception, wisdom, and insight that their unique minds have to offer. By empathetically entering their inner worlds one can appreciate the extraordinary resourcefulness of their minds, be grateful for their special talents, and enjoy their company more than ever.

Points to Keep in Mind

- Although traumatic experiences can govern the mind's original structure, skilled therapy can help a person reshape her mind.

- Various degrees of unification or cooperation are possible. A person with parts can decide which therapeutic goals seem most comfortable and helpful.

- Some parts wish to remain separate and can be advantageous in their separateness, while other parts will wish for integration once they can tell their memories or know that their separateness is no longer useful.

- From a mind in parts to a mind joined together is a major transition. The adjustment for the person and her intimates may require therapeutic help after the integration is complete.

- If people who have parts could disclose their compartmentalized minds without negative repercussions, they would be free to teach to singletons much that is fascinating and useful.

GLOSSARY

◉

CO-CONSCIOUSNESS The state of being conscious of the body's speech and actions but unable to control them. Co-consciousness is often described as the feeling of standing behind one's eyes or as watching one's actions on a screen. This term often implies the perception of closeness and belonging to the body even though unable to control it.

DEPERSONALIZATION The detachment of one's consciousness from the body so that one part of the mind is observing another part's experiences and actions. The observing part of the mind often describes this as the feeling of floating above the body and watching. *Depersonalization* and *co-consciousness* are terms similar in meaning, but depersonalization implies distance and alienation from the body so that the body is perceived as an object or as another person.

DISSOCIATION The existence of two or more separate parts of the personality. This state is specifically related to trauma.

HOST The part of the mind who has control of the body most of the time during a given time period. The given time period can be weeks, months, years, or a lifetime. Sometimes people with dissociated parts refer to the host as "the main person," "the outside person," "the core person," or "the presenter."

PART A dissociated part of the mind who develops an identity. Each part has her or his own memories, self-awareness, behaviors, emotions, functions, and perceptions. All parts together make up the whole personality.

PART FRAGMENT   A part of the mind quite limited in identity, with perhaps only one function or one emotion.

SINGLETON   A person who has a unified personality characterized by an uninterrupted continuation of consciousness, memory, control over the body, and sense of ownership: this is *my* intention, *my* thought, *my* voice, *my* action, *my* emotion, *my* body, *my* experience, and in future years these will be part of *my* memories.

SWITCHING   A shift in control of the body from one part of the mind to another.

Internet Resources

○

- **International Society for the Study of Dissociation** (issd.org)   Develops and promotes resources and responses to dissociation through training programs, conferences, online information, and the *Journal of Trauma and Dissociation*

- **Life Lessons from a Multiple Personality** (multiple-personality.com)   Offers one woman's publications and online ideas about using artwork and journal writing for self-understanding and healing

- **Many Voices** (manyvoicespress.com)   Publishes the newsletter *Many Voices* for people who experience trauma and dissociation and offers online resources

- **Mosaic Minds** (mosaicminds.org)   Online clearinghouse of information about dissociative identity disorder

- **National Alliance on Mental Illness** (NAMI; nami.org)   Mental health organization dedicated to improving the lives of people living with mental illness and their families' lives

- **Rape, Abuse, & Incest National Network** (RAINN; rainn.org)   Anti-sexual assault organization

- **The Sidran Institute** (sidran.org)   Traumatic stress education and advocacy

- **Survivors of Incest Anonymous** (siawso.org)   12-step self-help group for victims of child sexual abuse

- **Survivorship** (survivorship.org)   For victims of ritualistic abuse, mind control, and torture

- *The Wounded Healer Journal* (twhj.com)   For psychotherapists and others who have experienced trauma

ENDNOTES

◉

INTRODUCTION

1. These four questions are adapted from the *Diagnostic and Statistical Manual of Mental Disorders*, 4th ed., Text Revision (DSM-IV-TR), (Washington, DC: American Psychiatric Association, 2000), 529. Some researchers consider the criteria for dissociative identity disorder too narrow, and the classification is likely to change over the years due to newer research, as it has in the past. Concerning question four, many people who have dissociated identities originally attribute their signs of dissociation to substance abuse. Personal communication, Rhonda L. Sabo, July 2005.

2. Jane Wegscheider Hyman, *Women Living with Self Injury* (Philadelphia: Temple University Press, 1999).

3. Colin A. Ross, et al., "Multiple Personality Disorder: An Analysis of 236 Cases," *Canadian Journal of Psychiatry* 34 (June 1989): 416. In 2002, Ross confirmed that women make up 90 to 95 percent of people diagnosed as having DID or as having a related diagnosis called "dissociative disorder not otherwise specified." This figure is from the approximately three thousand admissions to his trauma program over nine years and conforms to all large studies of dissociative disorders. Colin A. Ross, "Sexual Orientation Conflict in the Dissociative Disorders," *Journal of Trauma and Dissociation* 3, no. 4 (2002): 137.

4. Rebecca M. Bolen, et al., "The Nature and Extent of Child Sexual Abuse," in *Home Truths About Child Sexual Abuse: Influencing Policy and Practice-A Reader,* ed. Catherine Itzin (New York: Routledge, 2000), 191.

5. Richard P. Kluft, "Dissociative Identity Disorder," in *Handbook of Dissociation: Theoretical, Empirical, and Clinical Perspectives,* eds. Larry K. Michelson and William J. Ray (New York: Plenum Press, 1996), 351.

6. Willie Langeland, et al., "Trauma and Dissociation in Treatment-Seeking Alcoholics: Towards a Resolution of Inconsistent Findings," *Comprehensive Psychiatry* 43, no. 3 (May/June 2002): 201.

7. Ibid.

8. Carol S. North, et al., *Multiple Personalities, Multiple Disorders: Psychiatric Classification and Media Influence* (New York: Oxford University Press, 1993), 53–54 (cites four studies); and personal communication Rhonda Sabo, July 2005.

9. E. L. Bliss, *Multiple Personalities, Allied Disorders and Hypnosis* (New York: Oxford University Press, 1986), cited in Stephen Kellett, "The Treatment of Dissociative Identity Disorder with Cognitive Analytic Therapy: Experimental Evidence of Sudden Gains," *Journal of Trauma and Dissociation* 6, no. 3 (2005): 56.

10. Carol S. North, et al., *Multiple Personalities, Multiple Disorders: Psychiatric Classification and Media Influence* (New York: Oxford University Press, 1993), 53–54 (cites four studies).

11. Richard P. Kluft, "Dissociative Identity Disorder," in *Handbook of Dissociation: Theoretical, Empirical, and Clinical Perspectives,* eds. Larry K. Michelson and William J. Ray (New York: Plenum Press, 1996), 350; J. Vanderlinden, et al., "Dissociative Experiences in the General Population in the Netherlands and Belgium: A Study With the Dissociative Questionnaire (DIS-Q)," *Dissociation* 4, no. 4 (1991), 180–184; J. Vanderlinden, et al., "Dissociation and Traumatic Experiences in the General Population of the Netherlands," *Hospital and Community Psychiatry* 44, no. 8 (1993): 786–788; Vedat Sar et al., "Prevalence of Dissociative Disorders Among Women in the General Population," article

in press, *Psychiatry Research*, 2006. Data from Hungary show 2.6 percent of the general population affected by DID. See J. Vanderlinden, et al., "Dissociative Symptoms in a Population Sample of Hungary," *Dissociation* 8, no. 4 (1995): 205–208.

12. Frank W. Putnam, *Diagnosis and Treatment of Multiple Personality Disorder* (New York: Guilford Press, 1989), 57.

13. The approximate figure of 2,683,953 women was calculated by taking 90 percent of 1 percent of the most recent (2006) projected total population of the United States, 298,217,000, according to the U.S. Bureau of the Census, U.S. Department of Commerce.

14. In 1989, even a specialist in the field complained of knowing "little about the day-to-day symptoms, experiences, and behavior of these unusual patients." Frank W. Putnam, *Diagnosis and Treatment of Multiple Personality Disorder* (New York: Guilford Press, 1989), 67. The literature since 1989 has brought more personal accounts but no studies on the lives of women who have DID. Therapists do not routinely collect data on their clients' experiences with mental health problems. See Francois Sainfort, et al., "Judgments of Quality of Life of Individuals with Severe Mental Disorders: Patient Self-Report vs. Provider Perspectives," *American Journal of Psychiatry* 153, no. 4 (April 1996): 498.

15. Regretting that many people know only the dramatic, horrifying situations in books and films about DID, Sandra J. Hocking writes, "What they don't see are the many multiples who have homes, families, jobs, and who live a fairly normal life. It doesn't make good copy." In Sandra J. Hocking and Company, *Living with Your Selves: A Survival Manual for People with Multiple Personalities* (Rockville, MD: Launch Press, 1992), 1.

16. This type currently falls under the category of "dissociative disorder not otherwise specified." It may be more prevalent than dissociative identity disorder. See, for example, Vedet Sar, et al., "Prevalence of Dissociative Disorders Among Women in the General Population," article in press, *Psychiatry Research*, 2006.

17. Some research suggests that, in fact, sadism is a strikingly frequent part of the abuse of people who have DID. See Frank W. Putnam, *Diagnosis and Treatment of Multiple Personality Disorder* (New York: Guilford Press, 1989), 49.

CHAPTER 1

1. Onno van der Hart, et al., "Dissociation: An Insufficiently Recognized Major Feature of Complex Posttraumatic Stress Disorder," *Journal of Traumatic Stress* 18, no. 5 (October 2005): 417.

2. Bessel A. van der Kolk and Onno van der Hart, "The Intrusive Past: The Flexibility of Memory and the Engraving of Trauma," *American Imago* 48 (1991): 446.

3. Panic attacks and the effects of an immediately preceding trauma such as a car accident are two examples of states of terror during which a person cannot absorb anything said to her or him. In "The Language of Dissociation," Na'ama Yehuda writes of the inability of traumatized children to process information presented in the classroom. *Journal of Trauma and Dissociation* 6, no. 1 (2005): 10 (cites two studies).

4. Pamela M. Cole and Frank W. Putnam, "Effect of Incest on Self and Social Functioning: A Developmental Psychopathology Perspective," *Journal of Consulting and Clinical Psychology* 60, no. 2 (1992): 179; and Colin A. Ross, "Epidemiology of Multiple Personality Disorder and Dissociation," *Psychiatric Clinics of North America* 14, no. 3 (September 1991): 505. The author based his figures on a series of 102 clients and considers these figures conservative.

5. For example, Canada, Holland, Puerto Rico, Turkey, and the USA. See Colin A. Ross, et al., "Abuse Histories in 102 Cases of Multiple Personality Disorder," *Canadian Journal of Psychiatry* 36 (March 1991): 99; Suzette Boon and Nel Draijer, *Multiple Personality Disorder in the Netherlands: A Study On Reliability and Validity of the Diagnosis* (Lisse, The Netherlands: Swets and Zeitlinger, 1993) as cited in Richard P. Kluft, "Dissociative Identity Disorder," *Handbook of Dissociation: The-*

oretical, Empirical, and Clinical Perspectives, eds. Larry K. Michelson and William J. Ray (New York: Plenum Press, 1996), 352; Alfonso Martinez-Taboas and Jose R. Rodriguez-Cay, "Case Study of a Puerto Rican Woman with Dissociative Identity Disorder," *Dissociation* 10, no. 3 (September 1997): 141; Vedet Sar, et al., "Prevalence of Dissociative Disorders Among Women in the General Population," article in press, *Psychiatry Research*, 2006; and Richard P. Kluft, et al., "Multiple Personality, Intrafamilial Abuse, and Family Psychiatry," *International Journal of Family Psychiatry*, 5, no. 1 (1984): 289.

6. Bessel A. van der Kolk, *Psychological Trauma* (Washington, DC: American Psychiatric Press, 1987), 16.

7. Martin H. Teicher and colleagues postulate that emotional abuse may prove to be an especially important factor in the development of dissociated identities, as they discuss in their funded grant application on the effects of emotional abuse, June 2005; and in Martin H. Teicher, M.D., Ph.D., et al., "Sticks, Stones and Hurtful Words: Combined Effects of Childhood Maltreatment Matter Most," manuscript submitted to the *American Journal of Psychiatry*, February 21, 2005. Ellert Nijenhuis and colleagues have found that although emotional neglect plays an important role, intense pain and threat to life from a person are the strongest predictors of physical signs of dissociation such as anaesthesia, or paralysis. Ellert R.S. Nijenhuis, et al., "Somatoform Dissociation, Reported Abuse and Animal Defence-Like Reactions," *Australian and New Zealand Journal of Psychiatry* (2004). Both research teams agree that experiencing multiple types of abuse seems to have the greatest impact of all.

8. Michael D. De Bellis, et al., "Developmental Traumatology Part II," *Biological Psychiatry* 45 (1999): 1276–1277; Martin H. Teicher, et al., "Childhood Neglect Is Associated with Reduced Corpus Callosum Area," *Biological Psychiatry* 56 (2004): 83; and Bessel A. van der Kolk, M.D. "The Neurobiology of Childhood Trauma and Abuse," *Child and Adolescent Psychiatric Clinics of North America* 12 (2003): 308, (cites studies from 1992 and 2002).

9. Ellert R.S. Nijenhuis, et al., "Degree of Somatoform and Psychological Dissociation in Dissociative Disorder Is Correlated with Reported Trauma," *Journal of Traumatic Stress* 11, no. 4 (1998): 711; and Martin H. Teicher, M.D., Ph.D., et al., "Sticks, Stones and Hurtful Words: Combined Effects of Childhood Maltreatment Matter Most," manuscript submitted to the *American Journal of Psychiatry*, February 21, 2005.

10. Martin H. Teicher, "Wounds That Time Won't Heal: The Neurobiology of Child Abuse," *Cerebrum: The Dana Forum on Brain Science* 2, no. 4 (Fall 2000): 55–57.

11. Ibid., 57–59. While several studies have linked a reduced left hippocampal volume to childhood abuse, other studies warn against concluding that abuse is the cause of the reduction. See Michael D. De Bellis, et al., "A Pilot Longitudinal Study of Hippocampal Volumes in Pediatric Maltreatment-Related Posttraumatic Stress Disorder," *Biological Psychiatry* 50 (2001): 305; J. Douglas Bremner, et al., "MRI and PET Study of Deficits in Hippocampal Structure and Function in Women with Childhood Sexual Abuse and Posttraumatic Stress Disorder," *American Journal of Psychiatry* 160, no. 5 (May 2003): 929; Cathy L. Pederson, et al., "Hippocampal Volume and Memory Performance in a Community-Based Sample of Women with Posttraumatic Stress Disorder Secondary to Child Abuse," *Journal of Traumatic Stress* 17 (February 2004): 37; and Marko Jelicic and Harald Merckelbach, "Traumatic Stress, Brain Changes, and Memory Deficits: A Critical Note," *The Journal of Nervous and Mental Disease* 192, no. 8 (August 2004): 548.

12. See Michael D. De Bellis, et al., "Developmental Traumatology Part II," *Biological Psychiatry* 45 (1999): 1276–1277; and Martin H. Teicher, et al., "Childhood Neglect Is Associated with Reduced Corpus Callosum Area," *Biological Psychiatry* 56 (2004): 83.

13. Murray B. Stein, et al., "Neuroanatomical and Neuroendocrine Correlates in Adulthood of Severe Sexual Abuse in Childhood," *American College of Neuropsychopharmacology Abstracts* 33 (1994): 53.

14. J. Douglas Bremner, et al., "MRI and PET Study of Deficits in Hippocampal Structure and Function in Women with Childhood Sexual Abuse and Posttraumatic Stress Disorder," *American Journal of Psychiatry* 160, no. 5 (May 2003): 929. However, Ellert Nijenhuis and Thomas Ehling found less volume in both the left and right hippocampus among people who had dissociative identity disorder or dissociative disorder not otherwise specified. They also found an association with hippocampal volume and a person's dissociative symptoms, posttraumatic stress symptoms, and reported exposure to potentially traumatizing events. Ellert Nijenhuis, personal communication, November 2005.

15. J. Douglas Bremner, et al., "MRI and PET Study of Deficits in Hippocampal Structure and Function in Women with Childhood Sexual Abuse and Posttraumatic Stress Disorder," *American Journal of Psychiatry* 160, no. 5 (May 2003): 929.

16. Onno van der Hart, et al., "Trauma-Related Dissociation: Conceptual Clarity Lost and Found," *Australian and New Zealand Journal of Psychiatry* 38 (2004): 908, cite P. H. Wolff, *The Development of Behavioral States and the Expression of Emotions in Early Infancy* (Chicago: University of Chicago Press, 1987).

17. Onno van der Hart, et al., "Trauma-Related Dissociation: Conceptual Clarity Lost and Found," *Australian and New Zealand Journal of Psychiatry* 38 (2004): 909, cite four studies.

18. Ellert R. S. Nijenhuis, et al., "The Emerging Psychobiology of Trauma-Related Dissociation and Dissociative Disorders," in *Biological Psychiatry*, ed. H. D'haenen, et al. (New York: John Wiley and Sons, Ltd., 2002), 1092.

19. Kathy Steele, et al., "Phase-Oriented Treatment of Structural Dissociation in Complex Traumatization: Overcoming Trauma-Related Phobias," *Journal of Trauma and Dissociation* 6, no. 3 (2005): 19.

20. Adapted from Cornelia B. Wilbur, "The Effect of Child Abuse on the Psyche," and Bennett G. Braun and Roberta G. Sachs, "The Development of Multiple Personality Disorder: Predisposing, Precipitating,

and Perpetuating Factors," in *Childhood Antecedents of Multiple Personality*, ed. Richard P. Kluft (Washington, DC: American Psychiatric Press, Inc., 1985): 27, 47, and 49; and Bennett G. Braun, "Towards a Theory of Multiple Personality and Other Dissociative Phenomena," in *The Psychiatric Clinics of North America, Symposium on Multiple Personality* 7, no. 1 (March 1984) (Philadelphia: W. B. Saunders, Co.): 173, 175.

21. See Bennett G. Braun and Roberta G. Sachs, "The Development of Multiple Personality Disorder: Predisposing, Precipitating, and Perpetuating Factors," in *Childhood Antecedents of Multiple Personality*, ed. Richard P. Kluft (Washington, DC: American Psychiatric Press, Inc., 1985): 47, 49; and Richard P. Kluft, "Dissociative Identity Disorder," in *Handbook of Dissociation: Theoretical, Empirical, and Clinical Perspectives*, eds. Larry K. Michelson and William J. Ray (New York: Plenum Press, 1996), 343.

22. E.R.S. Nijenhuis, *Somatoform Dissociation: Phenomena, Measurement, and Theoretical Issues* (New York: W.W. Norton & Company, 2004), 119. Researchers disagree on the possible importance of self-hypnosis. Eugene Bliss considers self-hypnosis a "primary mechanism" of DID. See "Multiple Personalities: A Report of Fourteen Cases with Implications for Schizophrenia and Hysteria," *Archives of General Psychiatry* 37 (December 1980): 1395. However, Ellert Nijenhuis points out a lack of solid evidence, and confusion as to what would count as dissociation as opposed to self-hypnosis. Personal communication, November 2005.

23. Jean L. Yates and William Nasby, "Dissociation, Affect, and Network Models of Memory: An Integrative Proposal," *Journal of Traumatic Stress* 6, no. 3 (1993): 312 (cite two studies).

24. This was the case for three of my interviewees: Ellie, when she was raped at knifepoint by a gang of men at age fourteen; Samantha, when at age forty-one she was suicidal; and Caroline, when at age thirty-seven her boss told her to take on a new type of work.

25. Jean L. Yates and William Nasby, "Dissociation, Affect, and Network Models of Memory: An Integrative Proposal," *Journal of Traumatic Stress*, 6, no. 3 (1993): 314.

26. Bessel A. van der Kolk, et al., "The History of Trauma in Psychiatry," *Psychiatric Clinics of North America* 17, no. 3 (September 1994): 585.

27. Bessel A. van der Kolk, "Trauma and Memory," in *Traumatic Stress: The Effects of Overwhelming Experience on Mind, Body, and Society*, ed. Bessel A. van der Kolk, et al. (New York: Guilford Press, 1996), 284–285, 287; and Ellert Nijenhuis, personal communication, November 2005.

28. Jennifer J. Freyd, et al., "Self-Reported Memory for Abuse Depends Upon Victim Perpetrator Relationship," *Journal of Trauma and Dissociation* 2, no. 3 (2001): 13–15. By 1919, the French researcher Pierre Janet had recognized that a person must be able to associate an experience with other events from life in order to assimilate it in memory as part of personal history. Cited by Bessel A. van der Kolk & Onno van der Hart in "The Intrusive Past: The Flexibility of Memory and the Engraving of Trauma," *American Imago* 48 (1991): 440.

29. Belinda Plattner, et al., "Pathways to Dissociation: Intrafamilial Versus Extrafamilial Trauma in Juvenile Delinquents," *The Journal of Nervous and Mental Disease* 191, no. 12 (December 2003): 786.

30. Kathryn A. Becker-Blease, et al., summarizes and supports this reasoning in "Preschoolers' Memory for Threatening Information Depends on Trauma History and Attentional Context: Implications for the Development of Dissociation," *Journal of Trauma and Dissociation* 5, no. 1 (2004): 114–115. Even being abused by someone close to her (as opposed to a stranger) decreases a child's likelihood of remembering the abuse as an adult. See Linda Meyer Williams, "Recall of Childhood Trauma: A Prospective Study of Women's Memories of Child Sexual Abuse," *Journal of Consulting and Clinical Psychology* 62, no. 6 (1994): 1172.

31. Onno van der Hart, et al., "Dissociation: An Insufficiently Recognized Major Feature of Complex Posttraumatic Stress Disorder," *Journal of Traumatic Stress* 18, no. 5 (October 2005), 416.

32. Bessel A. van der Kolk and Onno van der Hart, "The Intrusive Past: The Flexibility of Memory and the Engraving of Trauma," *American Imago* 48 (1991): 441–442.

33. This was temporarily the case for Reba, a participant in this study, who as her body's first identity "went deep inside" at age five but after therapy during young adulthood became able to function in the outside world once again, and perhaps permanently for Mary, whom I interviewed for *Women Living with Self-Injury* (Philadelphia: Temple University Press, 1999). At the time of the interview, Mary, her first identity's name, had remained submerged since childhood. The "Mary" I interviewed eventually introduced herself to me as Jennifer.

34. Bennett G. Braun, "Towards a Theory of Multiple Personality and Other Dissociative Phenomena," in *The Psychiatric Clinics of North America, Symposium on Multiple Personality* 7, no. 1 (March 1984) (Philadelphia: W. B. Saunders, Co.): 188.

35. Jean L. Yates and William Nasby, "Dissociation, Affect, and Network Models of Memory: An Integrative Proposal," *Journal of Traumatic Stress* 6, no. 3 (1993): 314.

36. Jean L. Yates and William Nasby, "Dissociation, Affect, and Network Models of Memory: An Integrative Proposal," *Journal of Traumatic Stress*, 6, no. 3 (1993): 314. Richard P. Kluft cites an average of thirteen to fifteen, while Colin A. Ross cites eight to nine as an average number of parts. See Richard P. Kluft, "Dissociative Identity Disorder," in *Handbook of Dissociation: Theoretical, Empirical, and Clinical Perspectives*, eds. Larry K. Michelson and William J. Ray (New York: Plenum Press, 1996), 340; and Colin A. Ross, et al., "Multiple Personality Disorder: An Analysis of 236 Cases" *Canadian Journal of Psychiatry*, 34 (June 1989): 417.

37. Richard P. Kluft, "Dissociative Identity Disorder," in *Handbook of Dissociation: Theoretical, Empirical, and Clinical Perspectives*, eds. Larry K.

Michelson and William J. Ray (New York: Plenum Press, 1996), 352 (cites six studies); and Frank W. Putnam, et al., "The Clinical Phenomenology of Multiple Personality Disorder: Review of 100 Recent Cases," *Journal of Clinical Psychiatry* 47, no. 6 (June 1986): 291–292 (cite their own and six other studies).

CHAPTER 2

1. The exception may be Gabbi, who, as the host, does not know what her mind's other parts do while she controls the body.
2. Changes in dominance between the left and right brain hemispheres may sometimes accompany the switching of parts and could help explain some of their diversity. See Polly Henninger, "Conditional Handedness: Handedness Changes in Multiple Personality Disordered Subject Reflect Shift in Hemispheric Dominance," *Consciousness and Cognition* 1 (1992): 265.
3. Frank W. Putnam, *Diagnosis and Treatment of Multiple Personality Disorder* (New York: Guilford Press, 1989), 112.
4. Shielagh R. Shusta-Hochberg, "Therapeutic Hazards of Treating Child Alters as Real Children in Dissociative Identity Disorder," *Journal of Trauma and Dissociation* 5, no. 1 (2004): 22.
5. In some cases, a therapist may name a part to make it more distinct and easier to work with. See Colin A. Ross, *Dissociative Identity Disorder: Diagnosis, Clinical Features, and Treatment of Multiple Personality* (New York: John Wiley and Sons, Inc., 1997), 311.
6. As does Joan Frances Casey when she relates needing only four to five hours of sleep at night. Joan Frances Casey with Lynn Wilson, *The Flock: The Autobiography of a Multiple Personality* (New York: Alfred A. Knopf, 1991), 246.
7. Colin A. Ross and Pam Gahan, "Cognitive Analysis of Multiple Personality Disorder," *American Journal of Psychotherapy* XLII (April 1988): 234.

8. Richard P. Kluft, "Clinical Presentations of Multiple Personality Disorder," *Psychiatric Clinics of North America* 14, no. 3 (September 1991): 611.

9. See, for example, Richard P. Kluft in "Dissociative Identity Disorder," in *Handbook of Dissociation: Theoretical, Empirical, and Clinical Perspectives,* eds. Larry K. Michelson and William J. Ray (New York: Plenum Press, 1996), 345–346; Frank W. Putnam, *Diagnosis and Treatment of Multiple Personality Disorder* (New York: Guilford Press, 1989), 106–114; and Colin A. Ross, *Dissociative Identity Disorder: Diagnosis, Clinical Features, and Treatment of Multiple Personality* (New York: John Wiley and Sons, Inc., 1997), 145–156.

10. Her name was changed to Cecelia when Samantha's second husband learned about Samantha's other identities and objected to Cecelia's former name.

11. The perpetrator is responsible for the abuse he or she inflicts. However, among women who have dissociated parts of the mind, the presence of sex-related parts may help explain why women abused as children are far more likely to be sexually assaulted as adults than those not abused. See M. Kay Jankowski, et al., "Parental Caring as a Possible Buffer Against Sexual Revictimization in Young Adult Survivors of Child Sexual Abuse," *Journal of Traumatic Stress* 15, no. 3 (June 2002): 235 (cite nine studies). For other explanations of abusive adult relationships after a childhood of abuse, see Chapter 7.

12. Frank W. Putnam, *Diagnosis and Treatment of Multiple Personality Disorder* (New York: Guilford Press, 1989), 111–112. The author refers only to the frequency of such parts at the workplace, while the majority of my interviewees also mention school.

13. Na'ama Yehuda, "The Language of Dissociation," *Journal of Trauma and Dissociation* 6, no. 1 (2005): 10.

14. See Colin A. Ross, *Dissociative Identity Disorder: Diagnosis, Clinical Features, and Treatment of Multiple Personality* (New York: John Wiley and Sons, Inc., 1997), 148–149; and Frank W. Putnam, *Diagnosis and Treatment of Multiple Personality Disorder* (New York: Guilford Press, 1989), 109–110.

15. Therapists who wish to work with a female client's male identity may find that he refuses to emerge if the client is wearing a dress. See Frank W. Putnam, *Diagnosis and Treatment of Multiple Personality Disorder* (New York: Guilford Press, 1989), 120.

16. Richard P. Kluft, "Body-Ego Integration in Dissociative Identity Disorder," in *Splintered Reflections: Images of the Body in Trauma*, eds. Jean Goodwin and Reina Attias (New York: Basic Books, 1999), 249.

17. Frank W. Putnam, *Diagnosis and Treatment of Multiple Personality Disorder* (New York: Guilford Press, 1989), 111–112.

18. Judy Dragon and Terry Popp, eds., *Multiple Journeys to One: Spiritual Stories of Integrating from Dissociative Identity Disorder* (Santa Rosa, California: Dancing Serpents Press, 1999), 134; and Robert B. Oxnam, *A Fractured Mind: My Life with Multiple Personality Disorder* (New York: Hyperion, 2005), 135–140.

19. Frank W. Putnam, *Diagnosis and Treatment of Multiple Personality Disorder* (New York: Guilford Press, 1989), 110.

20. Philip M. Coons, "Psychophysiologic Aspects of Multiple Personality Disorder: A Review," *Dissociation* 1 (March 1988): 50 (cites two studies).

21. Bennett G. Braun and Roberta G. Sachs, "The Development of Multiple Personality Disorder: Predisposing, Precipitating, and Perpetuating Factors," in *Childhood Antecedents of Multiple Personality*, ed. Richard P. Kluft (Washington, DC: American Psychiatric Press, Inc., 1985), 46.

22. Philip M. Coons, "Children of Parents with Multiple Personality Disorder," in *Childhood Antecedents of Multiple Personality*, ed. Richard P. Kluft (Washington, DC: American Psychiatric Press, Inc., 1985), 174–175.

23. Frank W. Putnam, et al., "The Clinical Phenomenology of Multiple Personality Disorder: Review of 100 Recent Cases," *Journal of Clinical Psychiatry* 47, no. 6 (June 1986): 288.

24. Some women have identities who rarely or never take over the body. Therefore, being switched is not a regular part of their experience.

25. Donald B. Beere considers apparent simultaneous control of the body by more than one part of the mind improbable and more likely to be rapid switching. See "Switching: Part 1, An Investigation Using Experimental Phenomenology," *Dissociation* 9, no. 1 (March 1996): 58.

26. Donald B. Beere, "Switching: Part 1, An Investigation Using Experimental Phenomenology," *Dissociation*, 9, no. 1 (March 1996): 56.

27. Philip M. Coons, "Multiple Personality Disorder: A Clinical Investigation of 50 Cases," *The Journal of Nervous and Mental Disease* 176, no. 9 (September 1988): 524. In her book *I'm Eve*, Chris Costner Sizemore describes her identity changes as often portended by severe headaches and accompanied by loss of bladder and bowel control, as though, briefly, unconsciousness had occurred. Chris Costner Sizemore and Elen Sain Pittillo (Garden City, NY: Doubleday and Company, Inc., 1977).

28. Philip M. Coons, "Psychophysiologic Aspects of Multiple Personality Disorder: A Review, *Dissociation* 1 (March 1988): 48 (cites three studies).

29. Richard J. Lowenstein, et al., "Experiential Sampling in the Study of Multiple Personality Disorder," *American Journal of Psychiatry* 144, no. 1 (January 1987): 23.

30. See Donald B. Beere, "Switching: Part 1, An Investigation Using Experimental Phenomenology," *Dissociation* 9, no. 1 (March 1996): 56.

31. This observation is supported by Donald B. Beere's study "Switching: Part 1, An Investigation Using Experimental Phenomenology," *Dissociation*, 9, no. 1 (March 1996): 55.

32. Frank W. Putnam, *Diagnosis and Treatment of Multiple Personality Disorder* (New York: Guilford Press, 1989), 62.

33. Eugene L. Bliss, "Multiple Personalities: A Report of 14 Cases with Implications for Schizophrenia and Hysteria," *Archives of General Psychiatry* 37 (December 1980): 1395; and Jean L. Yates and William Nasby, "Dissociation, Affect, and Network Models of Memory: An Integrative Proposal," *Journal of Traumatic Stress* 6, no. 3 (1993): 314.

34. Lisa D. Butler, et al., "Hypnotizability and Traumatic Experience: A Diathesis-Stress Model of Dissociative Symptomatology," *American Journal of Psychiatry* 153, no. 7 (July 1996 Festschrift Supplement): 43.

35. One published account describes part of a woman's mind telling her therapist about a combination of relaxation and concentration in first creating and activating another identity. See Eugene Bliss, "Multiple Personalities: A Report of Fourteen Cases with Implications for Schizophrenia and Hysteria," *Archives of General Psychiatry* 37 (December 1980): 1392.

36. Frank W. Putnam, "The Switch Process in Multiple Personality Disorder and Other State-Change Disorders," *Dissociation* 1 (March 1988): 27; and Philip M. Coons, "Psychophysiologic Aspects of Multiple Personality Disorder: A Review," *Dissociation* 1 (March 1988): 49.

37. Philip M. Coons, "Psychophysiologic Aspects of Multiple Personality Disorder: A Review, *Dissociation* 1 (March 1988): 49.

38. Philip M. Coons, "Children of Parents with Multiple Personality Disorder," in *Childhood Antecedents of Multiple Personality*, ed. Richard P. Kluft (Washington, DC: American Psychiatric Press, Inc., 1985), 175.

39. Richard P. Kluft, "The Natural History of Multiple Personality Disorder," in *Childhood Antecedents of Multiple Personality*, ed. Richard P. Kluft (Washington, DC: American Psychiatric Press, Inc., 1985), 202.

40. Frank W. Putnam, "The Switch Process in Multiple Personality Disorder and Other State-Change Disorders," *Dissociation*, 1 (March 1988): 28.

41. Frank W. Putnam, *Diagnosis & Treatment of Multiple Personality Disorder* (New York: Guilford Press, 1989), 118.

42. A. A. T. S. Reinders, et al., "Psychobiological Characteristics of DID: Neural, Physiologic, and Subjective Findings from a Symptom Provocation Study" (2005), manuscript submitted for publication; and A. A. T. S. Reinders, et al., "One Brain, Two Selves," *NeuroImage* 20 (2003): 2121.

43. Frances K. Grossman, personal communication, December 2004, based on Richard P. Kluft's observation.

CHAPTER 4

1. This was true for a woman called Carol, who recounts living in a meadow for thirty-eight years while other parts of her mind functioned as Carol. See Judy Dragon and Terry Popp, eds., *Multiple Journeys to One: Spiritual Stories of Integrating from Dissociative Identity Disorder* (Santa Rosa, CA: Dancing Serpents Press, 1999), 128–130.

2. This may prove to be the case for Mary, a forty-seven-year-old technology manager whom I interviewed for a previous project. Mary said that the original identity, called Mary, was "in the system" but did not function anymore. The "Mary" speaking to me then introduced herself as a part of Mary's mind called Jennifer. See Jane Wegscheider Hyman, *Women Living with Self-Injury* (Pittsburgh: Temple University Press, 1999), 20.

3. Donald B. Beere, "Switching: Part 1, An Investigation Using Experimental Phenomenology," *Dissociation* 9, no. 1 (March 1996): 56.

4. C. E., "The Internal Community Meeting—An Invaluable Tool," *Many Voices* (December 2001): 2.

CHAPTER 5

1. Frank W. Putnam, *Diagnosis and Treatment of Multiple Personality Disorder* (New York: Guilford Press, 1989), 126.

2. The identity in control may feel the impact of inner processes so that her mental state and/or her behavior are influenced. See Richard P. Kluft, "Clinical Presentations of Multiple Personality Disorder," *Psychiatric Clinics of North America* 14, no. 3 (September 1991): 612. This concept is discussed in Chapter 2.

3. An autobiographical account and some research has mentioned the workplace advantage of having parts whose specific focus is study

and/or work. See Bessel A. van der Kolk, "The Complexity of Adaptation to Trauma; Self-Regulation, Stimulus Discrimination, and Characterological Development," in *Traumatic Stress: The Effects of Overwhelming Experience on Mind, Body, and Society*, eds. Bessel A. van der Kolk, et al. (New York: Guilford Press, 1996), 192; Marlene Steinberg and Maxine Schnall, *The Stranger in the Mirror: Dissociation—the Hidden Epidemic* (New York: Cliff Street Books, 2000), 109; and Joan Frances Casey with Lynn Wilson, *The Flock: The Autobiography of a Multiple Personality* (New York: Alfred A. Knopf, 1991), 60, 246–247.

4. Overriding fatigue may be partly thanks to some parts' apparent ability to sleep while one or more others remain active, as discussed in Chapter 2.

5. Lynn W., "Work Life: What Do You Do with the Kids?" *Many Voices* (April 2003): 4.

6. Other researchers and people who have parts state that parts can cause work difficulties or job losses. See Frank W. Putnam, *Diagnosis and Treatment of Multiple Personality Disorder* (New York: Guilford Press, 1989), 207; Marlene Steinberg and Maxine Schnall, *The Stranger in the Mirror: Dissociation—the Hidden Epidemic* (New York: Cliff Street Books, 2000), 109; Chris Costner Sizemore and Elen Sain Pittillo, *I'm Eve* (Garden City, NY: Doubleday and Company, Inc., 1977), 276–280; and Daniel Keyes, *The Minds of Billy Milligan* (New York: Random House, Inc., 1981), 209, 217, 276.

7. Lucy, a social worker, has felt the urge to abuse the adolescents in her care, a "familiar, uncomfortable feeling" that frightened Lucy. She has always stopped the urge, and says that she is certain that her clients are safe with her. Lucy discussed the matter with her therapist, who agreed that Lucy would never act on such feelings. Richard P. Kluft reports that two female physicians who were his clients feared failing their own patients if they were upset by painful memories discussed in therapy. In "High Functioning Multiple Personality Patients," *The Journal of Nervous and Mental Disease* 174, no. 12 (1986): 726.

CHAPTER 7

1. Frank W. Putnam, et al., "The Clinical Phenomenology of Multiple Personality Disorder: Review of 100 Recent Cases," *Journal of Clinical Psychiatry* 47 (June 1986): 289.

2. Colin A. Ross, "Sexual Orientation Conflict in the Dissociative Disorders," *Journal of Trauma and Dissociation* 3, no. 4 (2002): 142; and Frank W. Putnam, *Diagnosis and Treatment of Multiple Personality Disorder* (New York: Guilford Press, 1989), 111.

3. See James A. Chu, *Rebuilding Shattered Lives: The Responsible Treatment of Complex Post-Traumatic and Dissociative Disorders* (New York: John Wiley and Sons, Inc., 1998), 103, 106.

4. Richard P. Kluft, et al., say that such involvements are "not unusual" among people who have DID. In "Multiple Personality, Intrafamilial Abuse, and Family Psychiatry," *International Journal of Family Psychiatry* 5, no. 1 (1984): 297.

5. See James A. Chu, *Rebuilding Shattered Lives: The Responsible Treatment of Complex Post-Traumatic and Dissociative Disorders* (New York: John Wiley and Sons, Inc., 1998), 103, 106. (For the statement on emotional bonding, Chu cites D. Dutton and S. L. Painter, "Traumatic Bonding: The Development of Emotional Attachments in Battered Women and Other Relationships of Intermittent Abuse," *Victimology* 6 (1981): 139–155.)

6. Elizabeth Bowman, personal communication, August 2005.

7. Anne P. DePrince, "Social Cognition and Revictimization Risk," *Journal of Trauma and Dissociation* 6, no. 1 (2005): 125.

8. James A. Chu, *Rebuilding Shattered Lives: The Responsible Treatment of Complex Post-Traumatic and Dissociative Disorders* (New York: John Wiley and Sons, Inc., 1998), 106.

9. "Tonic Immobility" is a survival tactic among mammals. See H. Stefan Bracha, "Freeze, Flight, Fight, Fright, Faint: Adaptationist Perspectives on the Acute Stress Response Spectrum," *CNS Spectrums* 9, no. 9 (September 2004): 680.

CHAPTER 8

1. For example, see Chapters 7 and 26 in *Cameron West, First Person Plural: My Life as a Multiple* (New York: Hyperion, 1999).

2. Frank W. Putnam, *Diagnosis and Treatment of Multiple Personality Disorder* (New York: Guilford Press, 1989), 207; and Bessel A. van der Kolk, et al., *Traumatic Stress: The Effects of Overwhelming Experience on Mind, Body, and Society* (New York: Guilford Press, 1996), 192.

3. Elizabeth S. Bowman, personal communication, August 2005.

4. These three points are the findings of Richard P. Kluft, et al., "Multiple Personality, Intrafamilial Abuse, and Family Psychiatry," *International Journal of Family Psychiatry* 5, no. 1 (1984): 297–298. Kluft and his colleagues state that in their experience, "over 90 percent of the relationships in which the optimal stance is taken fare well, but a substantial number of those in which less constructive stances prevail deteriorate and come to an end."

5. Recounted by Richard P. Kluft about a mother in his study "The Parental Fitness of Mothers with Multiple Personality Disorder: A Preliminary Study," *Child Abuse and Neglect* 11 (1987): 277.

6. Richard P. Kluft, et al., "Multiple Personality, Intrafamilial Abuse, and Family Psychiatry," *International Journal of Family Psychiatry* 5, no. 1 (1984): 297.

7. Colin A. Ross has found conflict about sexuality and sexual orientation to be "universal in complex multiple personality disorder." *Multiple Personality Disorder: Diagnosis, Clinical Features, and Treatment of Multiple Personality* (New York: John Wiley and Sons, Inc., 1989), 118.

8. Elizabeth Bowman, personal communication, August 2005.

9. Richard P. Kluft, et al., "Multiple Personality, Intrafamilial Abuse, and Family Psychiatry," *International Journal of Family Psychiatry* 5, no. 1 (1984): 297.

10. It is unclear how much Samantha's first husband knew.

11. Richard P. Kluft, et al., "Multiple Personality, Intrafamilial Abuse, and Family Psychiatry," *International Journal of Family Psychiatry* 5, no. 1 (1984): 297.

CHAPTER 9

1. See Cameron West, *First Person Plural: My Life as a Multiple* (New York: Hyperion, 1999), 193–194, 313.

2. See Barry M. Cohen, et al., eds., *Multiple Personality Disorder from the Inside Out* (Lutherville, MD: Sidran Press, 1991), 41, 49, 189; Judy Dragon and Terry Popp, eds., *Multiple Journeys to One: Spiritual Stories of Integrating from Dissociative Identity Disorder* (Santa Rosa, CA: Dancing Serpents Press, 1999), 31, 32, 141, 199; and Rachel Downing, "Reflections on Being a Parent with DID," *Many Voices* (June 2003): 7.

3. Lynn R. Benjamin, et al., "Dissociative Mothers' Subjective Experience of Parenting," *Child Abuse and Neglect* 20, no. 10 (1996): 939.

4. Richard P. Kluft, "The Parental Fitness of Mothers with Multiple Personality Disorder: A Preliminary Study," *Child Abuse and Neglect* 11 (1987): 273–274.

5. Ibid., 273; and Colin A. Ross, et al., "Multiple Personality Disorder: An Analysis of 236 Cases," *Canadian Journal of Psychiatry* 34 (June 1989): 416.

6. David Singh Narang and Josefina M. Contreras, "Dissociation as a Mediator Between Child Abuse History and Adult Abuse Potential," *Child Abuse and Neglect* 24, no. 5 (2000): 660.

7. Delphine Collin-Vezina, et al., "The Role of Depression and Dissociation in the Link Between Childhood Sexual Abuse and Later Parental Practices," *Journal of Trauma and Dissociation* 6, no. 1 (2005): 89.

8. Frank W. Putnam, *Diagnosis and Treatment of Multiple Personality Disorder* (New York: Guilford Press, 1989), 105.

9. See Richard P. Kluft's example of two mothers in his study "The Parental Fitness of Mothers with Multiple Personality Disorder: A Preliminary Study," *Child Abuse and Neglect* 11 (1987): 277.

10. Colin A. Ross, "Sexual Orientation Conflict in the Dissociative Disorders," *Journal of Trauma and Dissociation* 3, no. 4 (2002): 142.

11. This was the case of a woman who had a teenage part attracted to the woman's fourteen-year-old son, as recounted in Richard P. Kluft, "The

Parental Fitness of Mothers with Multiple Personality Disorder: A Preliminary Study," *Child Abuse and Neglect* 11 (1987): 278.

12. Lynn R. Benjamin and Robert Benjamin, "An Overview of Family Treatment in Dissociative Disorders," *Dissociation* 5, no. 4 (December 1992): 238.

13. Philip M. Coons, "Children of Parents with Multiple Personality Disorder," in *Childhood Antecedents of Multiple Personality*, ed. Richard P. Kluft (Washington, DC: American Psychiatric Press, 1985), 163.

14. Lynn R. Benjamin and Robert Benjamin, "An Overview of Family Treatment in Dissociative Disorders," *Dissociation* 5, no. 4 (December 1992): 238.

15. International Society for the Study of Dissociation [Members of the Guidelines Revision Task Force], "Guidelines for Treating Dissociative Identity Disorder in Adults (2005)," *Journal of Trauma & Dissociation* 6, no. 4 (2005): 136.

16. Richard P. Kluft, "The Parental Fitness of Mothers with Multiple Personality Disorder: A Preliminary Study," *Child Abuse and Neglect* 11 (1987): 273.

17. Lynn R. Benjamin and Robert Benjamin have found these same problems among their clients who come to them for family therapy related to DID. See "An Overview of Family Treatment in Dissociative Disorders," *Dissociation* 5, no. 4 (December 1992): 238.

18. In their comparison study "Predicting Rejection of Her Infant from Mother's Representation of Her Own Experiences," *Child Abuse and Neglect* 8 (1984): 203–217, M. Main and R. Goldwyn found that nonabusive mothers recognized the effects their own childhood abuse had on them and the potential harm such abuse could have on their own children. In contrast, abusive mothers did not associate their feelings with any memories they had and seemed to lack an understanding of the relationship between their own childhood experiences and their current childcare practices. As cited in Byron Egeland, et al., "Breaking the Cycle of Abuse, *Child Development* 59 (1988): 1087.

19. Psychologist Martha Stout has found that those clients with DID fare best who feel strong responsibility for someone or something, as stated in *The Myth of Sanity: Divided Consciousness and the Promise of Awareness* (New York: Viking, 2001), 210–211.

CHAPTER 10

1. Rose would find her assumption confirmed by at least one woman who used exactly the same analogy in writing about her experience of "getting better." "In losing a structure that had sustained me for most of my sixty years, I . . . felt like an immigrant in a foreign country. I didn't know the customs, the culture, or the rules of engagement." From Laura/Vivian, "New Landscape: Support Group for Almost-Betters in New York," *Many Voices* (April 2005): 6.
2. Richard P. Kluft, untitled article on spontaneous integration, "Therapist's Page," *Many Voices* (April 2000): 6.
3. See Thea, "Thoughts on Integration," *Many Voices* (August 2003): 10.
4. Colin A. Ross, personal communication, May 2005.
5. Reba, a nurse, who critiqued this chapter, confirmed with a comment in the margin the importance of Ellie's strategy of planning ahead. Reba wrote, "This is very important to do! We do this too, especially for exams (pap tests, mammograms, etc.). Either I, (Reba), or Circle is at the appointment and the kids go into the safe room until we get home."
6. Judy Dragon and Terry Popp, eds., *Multiple Journeys to One: Spiritual Stories of Integrating from Dissociative Identity Disorder* (Santa Rosa, CA: Dancing Serpents Press, 1999), 67.
7. Richard P. Kluft, "The Postunification Treatment of Multiple Personality Disorder: First Findings," *American Journal of Psychotherapy* XLII, no. 2 (April 1988): 215 (cites three studies); and Colin A. Ross, *Dissociative Identity Disorder: Diagnosis, Clinical Features, and Treatment of Multiple Personality* (New York: John Wiley and Sons, Inc., 1997), 378.

8. Richard P. Kluft, "The Postunification Treatment of Multiple Personality Disorder: First Findings," *American Journal of Psychotherapy* XLII, no. 2 (April 1988): 216; and Richard P. Kluft, untitled article on spontaneous integration, "Therapist's Page," *Many Voices* (April 2000): 6.

9. Richard Kluft, "On Treating the Older Patient with Multiple Personality Disorder: 'Race Against Time' or 'Make Haste Slowly?'" *American Journal of Clinical Hypnosis* 30, no. 4 (April 1988): 259.

10. Ibid., 258.

11. Richard P. Kluft, untitled article on spontaneous integration, "Therapist's Page," *Many Voices* (April 2000): 7.

12. See Judy Dragon and Terry Popp, eds., *Multiple Journeys to One: Spiritual Stories of Integrating from Dissociative Identity Disorder* (Santa Rosa, CA: Dancing Serpents Press, 1999), 14, 133; and Colin A. Ross, *Dissociative Identity Disorder: Diagnosis, Clinical Features, and Treatment of Multiple Personality* (New York: John Wiley and Sons, Inc., 1997), 376.

13. Judy Dragon and Terry Popp, ed., *Multiple Journeys to One: Spiritual Stories of Integrating from Dissociative Identity Disorder* (Santa Rosa, CA: Dancing Serpents Press, 1999), 28, 46.

14. Colin A. Ross, M.D., *Dissociative Identity Disorder: Diagnosis, Clinical Features, and Treatment of Multiple Personality* (New York: John Wiley & Sons, Inc., 1997), 376.

15. "[W]e have come together in the presence of God to witness and proclaim the joining together of this man and this woman in marriage," etc. All such references probably evolved from Matthew 19:6: "Those whom God hath joined together let no man put asunder."

16. For an example of such verbal guidance see Colin A. Ross *Dissociative Identity Disorder: Diagnosis, Clinical Features, and Treatment of Multiple Personality* (New York: John Wiley and Sons, Inc., 1997), 376–377.

17. Sandra J. Hocking and Company, *Living with Your Selves: A Survival Manual for People with Multiple Personalities* (Rockville, MD: Launch Press, 1992), 4.

18. Such a variety of responses to integration are depicted in Chris Cost-
    ner Sizemore, *A Mind of My Own* (New York: William Morrow and
    Company, Inc., 1989), 49; Judy Dragon and Terry Popp, eds., *Multi-
    ple Journeys to One: Spiritual Stories of Integrating from Dissociative Iden-
    tity Disorder* (Santa Rosa, CA: Dancing Serpents Press, 1999), 23,
    68–71; Katrina, "Integration," *Many Voices* (April 2000): 3; Laura,
    "Learning to Navigate in a New Landscape: Difficulties of Getting Bet-
    ter," *Many Voices* (April 2004): 6–9; and Laura/Vivian, "New Land-
    scape: Support Group for Almost-Betters in New York," *Many Voices*
    (April 2005): 6.

19. Richard P. Kluft, "The Postunification Treatment of Multiple Person-
    ality Disorder: First Findings," *American Journal of Psychotherapy* XLII,
    no. 2 (April 1988): 225.

20. Chris Costner Sizemore and Elen Sain Pittillo, *I'm Eve* (Garden City,
    NY: Doubleday and Company, Inc., 1977), 4.

21. Judy Dragon and Terry Popp, eds., *Multiple Journeys to One: Spiritual
    Stories of Integrating from Dissociative Identity Disorder* (Santa Rosa, CA:
    Dancing Serpents Press, 1999), 91; and Chris Costner Sizemore, *A
    Mind of My Own* (New York: William Morrow and Company, Inc.,
    1989), 32, 178.

22. *Harmonization* is the term some people prefer in describing their goal.
    See Tammy Colleen Whitman and Susan C. Shore, *The Multiple's
    Guide to Harmonized Family Living: A Healthy Alternative (or Prelude)
    to Integration* (Marina Del Rey, CA: Artistic Endeavors Publishing,
    1994), 11.

INDEX

◉

Abortions, 53, 70, 76, 155, 163
Abuse. *See* Childhood abuse; Emotional
   abuse; Intellectual abuse; Physical
   abuse; Sexual abuse; Sexual
   partnerships, abusive
ADHD, 215
Administrators (parts), 50
Adolescent parts, 46, 87, 149–64, 242.
   See also Child parts; Sex
   integration and, 233–34
   parenting and, 218
   typical functions of, 43
   work and, 108, 129
Adult parts
   older than host, 49, 245–46
   typical functions of, 43
   work and, 115, 128–29, 130, 133
Age. *See also* Adolescent parts; Adult
   parts; Child parts
   formation of new parts and, 34
   self-perception of, 44–45, 159, 199,
     223
   of study participants, 7
   switching frequency and, 230
   trauma-induced freezing of, 33
Alcohol use/abuse, 2, 4, 196, 205, 207,
   214, 215
Allergies, 77
Alters
   Ellie's name for parts, 58, 209
   reason for not using term in study, 14

Amnesia. *See* Memory lapses
Amy (part of Reba), 231
Andi (part of Reba), 47
Angel (part of Reba), 47
Angie (part of Reba), 231
Annie (part of Reba), 230, 231–32, 235
Anorexia nervosa, 40, 215
Aristocrat, The (part of Ruth), 103

Barbara (host), 37, 39–40, 42, 43, 47,
   48–49, 54, 247. *See also* Chore
   Boy; Day Girl, The; Dog Girl;
   GaGa; Math Girl; Night Girl, The;
   OwOw; Slugger; Slut Girl;
   Working Girl
   appreciation of parts, 238–40, 241,
     243
   description of, 8
   on disclosure, 131–32
   dwelling places for parts, 102, 104
   on integration, 221, 226, 227, 228
   organization of parts, 82
   self-injury in, 52
   self-presentation by, 44
   sex and, 46, 157–58, 160, 161
   sexual abuse of, 157
   switching in, 60, 63
   work and, 48, 113, 127, 128, 129,
     131–32, 243
Beckilynn (part of Reba), 47
Belgium, DID prevalence in, 6

279

About the Author

◉

Jane W. Hyman grew up in Dallas, Texas. As a young adult, she moved to Vienna, Austria, where she lived for seventeen years. There she collaborated with a small group of women to establish a women's center and a feminist women's magazine for which she occasionally wrote articles. With a friend, she started a women's bookstore and café called *Frauenzimmer*, the first of its kind in Vienna. It was there that she met two women from the Boston Women's Health Book Collective who had come to Vienna to help Austrian and German women start a German-language edition of *Our Bodies, Ourselves*. This fortuitous meeting sparked a collaboration in the U.S. on book projects and eventually a career as an independent researcher and writer on women's health.

Hyman is the author of *Women Living with Self-Injury* and *The Light Book* and, with the late Esther Rome, of *Sacrificing Our Selves for Love*. She is also a co-author of *Ourselves, Growing Older* and *The New Our Bodies, Ourselves*. Over time, the focus of her work shifted from physical health to mental health partly through her own experiences with obsessive-compulsive disorder and depression. As important pastimes, she enjoys reading in English and German, dusting off her French, and playing the viola da gamba and recorder with other amateur musicians.

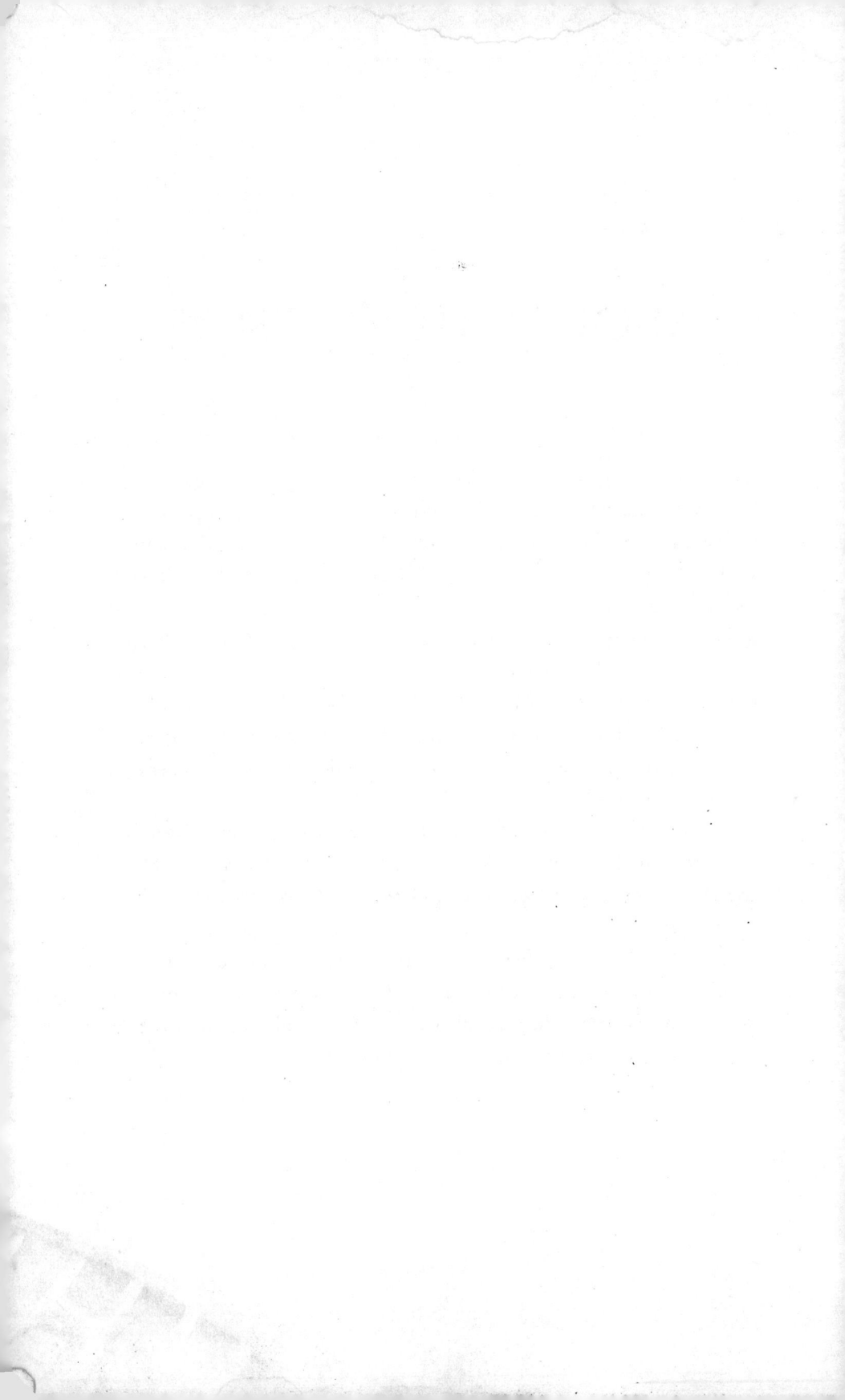